EYE INJURIES

An illustrated guide

EYE INJURIES

An illustrated guide

Elizabeth M. Eagling MB, BS, FRCS

Consultant Ophthalmic Surgeon
Birmingham & Midland Eye Hospital
and Selly Oak Hospital
Birmingham, UK

Michael J. Roper–Hall MB, ChM, FRCS

Consultant Ophthalmic Surgeon
Birmingham & Midland Eye Hospital
and Queen Elizabeth Hospital
Birmingham, UK

 J.B. Lippincott Company Philadelphia

Gower Medical Publishing London · New York

Distribution

UK
Butterworth & Co. (Publishers) Ltd.
Borough Green
Sevenoaks
Kent TN15 8PH, UK

USA & Canada
J.B. Lippincott Company
East Washington Square
Philadelphia
PA 10105, USA

Japan
Nishimura Co., Ltd.
1-754-39 Asahimachi-dori
Niigata-Shi 951, Japan

British Library Cataloguing in Publication Data
Eagling, Elizabeth M.
Eye injuries: an illustrated guide.
1. Eye – Wounds and injuries
I. Title   II. Roper–Hall, M.J.
617.7'13   RE831

Library of Congress Catalog Card Number 86-80146

ISBN: 0–906923–32–8 (Gower)
0–397–58301–X (Lippincott)

Project Editors: Helen Hadjidimitriadou
Fiona Lake

Design: Eva Bozser

Illustration: Pam Corfield
Jeremy Cort

Typeset by Informat in Linotype Bembo and Helvetica
Origination in Hong Kong by Imago Publishing Ltd.
Printed in Hong Kong by Mandarin Offset Intl. Ltd.

Preface

Fifty years ago of the management of penetrating eye injuries was dominated by the fear of sympathetic ophthalmitis; patients frequently presented several days after injury, and the incidence of sympathetic ophthalmitis was high. Once established, there was no effective treatment and blindness often resulted.

At that time ophthalmologists were beginning to realise that tissue incarceration and persisting intraocular inflammation increased the risk of sympathetic ophthalmitis. Over the years advanced techniques of repair have improved the outcome, and our thoughts are no longer dominated by the fear of sympathetic inflammation. Surgical repair has become more precise with the use of the operating microscope, atraumatic needles and fine suture material, while the harmful effect of infection and inflammation can largely be controlled by modern drug therapy.

Our present knowledge has come from careful evaluation of each new advance; in the last decade exciting possibilities have opened up with the development of machines capable of removing both damaged lens and vitreous through very small incisions, while modern contact lens and intraocular implants have improved the outcome of a traumatic cataract.

This book is intended as a practical guide to the early management of ophthalmic injuries, on which the outcome so often depends. It has been primarily written for ophthalmologists in training, but we hope it will have a wider appeal, both to practising ophthalmologists who may not see major eye injuries very frequently, and to surgeons in other disciplines dealing with facial and head injuries.

Acknowledgements

Our thanks to all staff at the Birmingham and Midland Eye Hospital and many other colleagues who have helped to provide illustrations, to Mr A.R. Groves and Mr. J.P. Gowar for their help on facial burns, and to Mr. M.J.C. Wake for his advice and illustrations of orbital injuries.

Dedicated to our colleagues

Contents

1

In the Accident Department

THE ASSESSMENT OF EYE INJURIES

The recognition and preliminary assessment of eye injuries is the responsibility of the Casualty Officer. As in all medical disciplines, this involves taking a detailed history, conducting an examination, and arranging special investigations.

History

A detailed history can help predict the type of damage to be expected. Certain common patterns are observed: for example, a patient presenting with a history of something hitting his eye after using a hammer and chisel has an intraocular foreign body until proven otherwise. If the patient also describes black cobwebs ('floaters') affecting his vision, then the foreign body must be located in the posterior part of the globe, because a small vitreous haemorrhage has occurred. This is the commonest location of an intraocular foreign body.

The history of hammering steel on steel indicates that this foreign body is magnetic and therefore amenable to surgical removal with an electromagnet.

This is one example of how the history can predict the extent of the problem following an injury, and help in planning the management.

History should include:

1. A detailed description of how the eye injury was caused, and subsequent symptoms.
2. Details of other injuries.
3. First–aid treatment given.
4. Previous history of eye disease.
5. General medical history.
6. Immune status and known allergies.

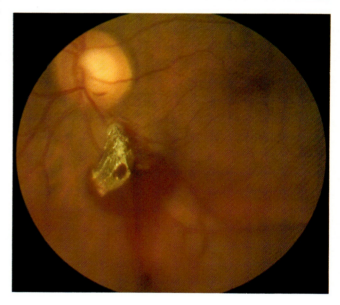

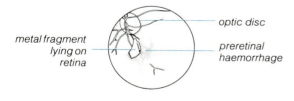

Fig.1.1 A foreign body impacted on the retina.

The history may not be reliable in children, and even apparently trivial injuries must be treated seriously; a commonly missed injury results from falling onto a pointed object: externally the entry wound may be very small, but such injuries can damage the optic nerve or penetrate the roof of the orbit and lead to serious complications. Similar injuries may occur in sport, and in this example the affected eye was blinded by a finger poked in the eye in a rugby scrum.

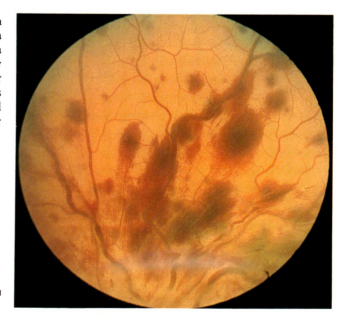

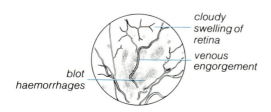

Fig.1.2 Fundus appearance shows retinal infarction from optic nerve evulsion after a finger was poked in the eye.

When taking the history, ask what first-aid treatment has been given: for chemical burns it is helpful to know how quickly and how effectively the eyes have been irrigated. In injuries from a dart or other sharply pointed object, enquire whether the object fell out of the eye or whether it had to be pulled out; if the latter, a double perforation must be suspected. In accidents at work involving broken tools or wire, ask if these have been inspected; if any part is missing, see if it can be accounted for: fragments may hit the eye and fall away, or they may penetrate and remain impacted in the wound.

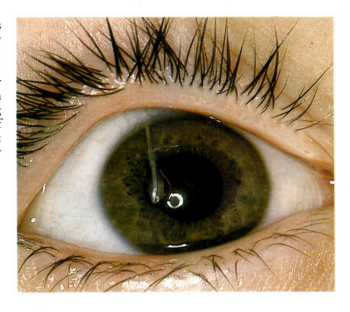

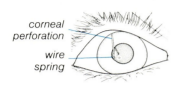

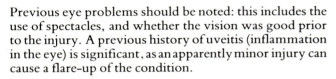

Fig.1.3 A piece of wire causing a perforating injury.

Previous eye problems should be noted: this includes the use of spectacles, and whether the vision was good prior to the injury. A previous history of uveitis (inflammation in the eye) is significant, as an apparently minor injury can cause a flare-up of the condition.

Details of any other injuries should be noted, together with a general medical history including regular medication, known drug allergies, and whether immunised against tetanus.

Examination

General supportive measures

Many eye injuries are painful and the first step is to place the patient in a recumbent position and establish the extent of the injuries. When there is a possibility of multiple injuries particular attention must be paid to head, chest and abdominal injuries; treatment of any life-threatening condition must have priority.

Facial lacerations may bleed profusely, and one or two temporary sutures may be required to staunch the bleeding. Marked oedema of the eyelids may be present following a contusion injury or chemical burn, and this may make examination difficult; a general anaesthetic may be necessary to exclude an underlying rupture of the

globe, or to perform adequate irrigation for a chemical burn.

Any injury resulting in a laceration should have tetanus prophylaxis in addition to surgical toilet. In clean wounds less than six hours old, a booster or full course of tetanus toxoid is given according to the immune status; in all other wounds, human tetanus immunoglobulin is required in addition to tetanus toxoid if the patient is not immunised against tetanus or the last booster was over ten years ago. If giving human tetanus immunoglobulin, adrenaline 0.5 - 1.0 mg I.M. must be available in case of anaphylaxis.

Assessment of vision

This is a very important part of the initial examination; each eye is tested separately with a light sterile dressing or card occluding the other eye. Even in major eye injuries the ability to perceive light and to tell its direction when tested from each quadrant should be recorded.

Unless there is a risk of aggravating an extensive perforating injury, testing should proceed to establish the best level of vision; if hand movements can be perceived, the ability to count fingers is tested at one metre, then formal testing using a Snellen test type is performed.

Glasses may have been broken in the accident, and in less severe injuries the test is repeated using a pin-hole lens to overcome any refractive error.

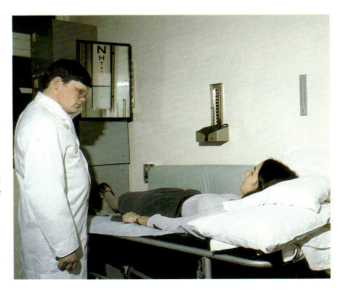

Fig.1.4 The emergency room should be arranged so that a recumbent patient can see an illuminated test type reflected in a suitably positioned mirror.

Simple eye examination: using focal illumination

All procedures should first be explained to the patient and the manoeuvres carried out in a gentle fashion to minimise exacerbating any underlying injury.

After inspecting the eyelids for signs of bruising or laceration, the eye itself is examined by gently retracting the upper lid using a sterile gauze swab and instructing the patient to keep both eyes open. A narrow beam of light from a pen torch is used to illuminate the eye.

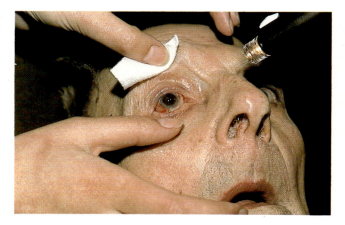

Fig.1.5   Examining an injured eye.

If active bleeding is apparent from beneath the eyelids, a major penetrating injury is present and the eye should not be disturbed further until repair can be arranged. Otherwise the examination proceeds as follows:

The cornea and anterior chamber are first checked for a laceration or bleeding. Shallowness of the anterior chamber suggests a leaking wound; this is assessed by comparing the depth of the anterior chamber in the injured eye and unaffected eye. In this example there is a corneal laceration, with a flat anterior chamber and traumatic cataract.

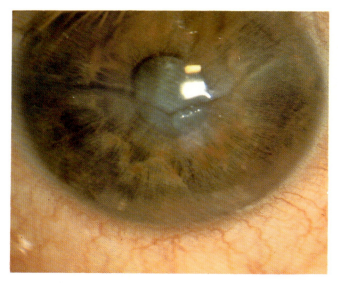

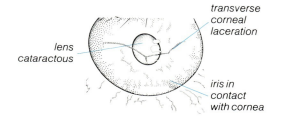

Fig.1.6   Corneal laceration with a flat anterior chamber.

A pear-shaped distortion of the pupil indicates prolapse of the iris into a wound; a knuckle of iris tissue may be visible externally.

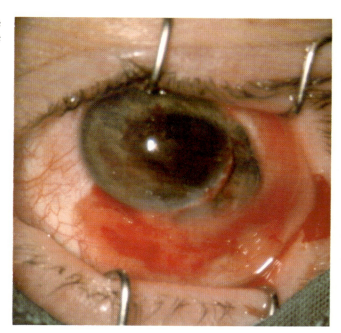

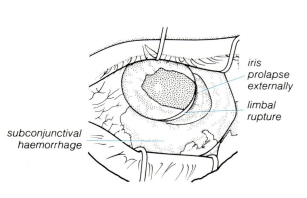

Fig.1.7   Iris prolapse after a perforating injury.

An irregular pupil is also seen after contusion; in the absence of a laceration, the anterior chamber is usually of normal depth, but blood may be present forming a fluid level below. This is known as an hyphaema.

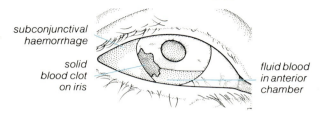

subconjunctival haemorrhage

solid blood clot on iris

fluid blood in anterior chamber

Fig.1.8 Bleeding into the anterior chamber after a blunt injury.

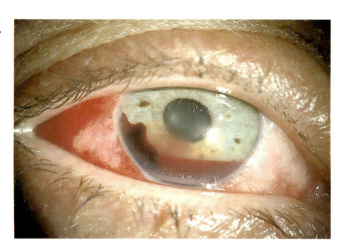

The sclera is then checked by examining each quadrant in turn, instructing the patient to look in the appropriate direction; a scleral perforation may be obscured by haemorrhage under the conjunctiva, but any sign of dark pigment indicates prolapse of the underlying tissues and confirms a perforating injury. Prolapse of vitreous gel may be visible on the surface.

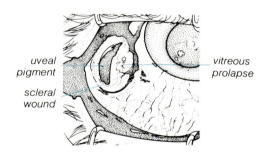

uveal pigment

scleral wound

vitreous prolapse

Fig.1.9 Scleral laceration with vitreous prolapse.

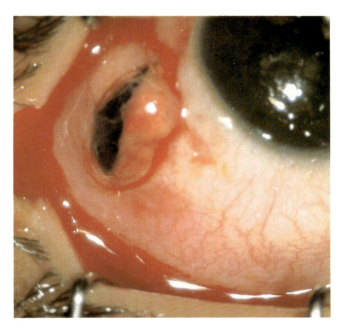

Simple eye examination: using the direct ophthalmoscope

If there is no major perforating injury, the structures situated more posteriorly in the eye can be examined with the direct ophthalmoscope. If the eye is viewed through the ophthalmoscope from three feet away with the patient looking at the light, a red glow emerges through the pupil from light reflected internally. Any opacity that disturbs the transmission of light (such as a corneal laceration or damage to the lens) will show up as a dark shadow against the red reflex. In this example, the track of a foreign body through the lens of the eye is seen against the red reflex.

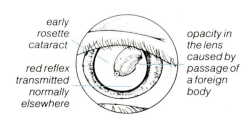

early rosette cataract

red reflex transmitted normally elsewhere

opacity in the lens caused by passage of a foreign body

Fig.1.10 Lens damage seen against the red reflex.

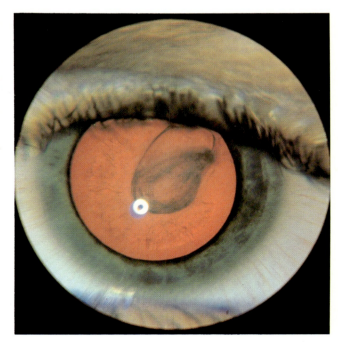

1.5

If there is no opacity obscuring the view, the ophthalmoscope is brought close to the eye to examine the posterior structures. The examination commences with a +10 lens in position, which focuses on the anterior vitreous; by reducing the strength of the lens in the ophthalmoscope the focus is directed posteriorly until the retina can be clearly seen.

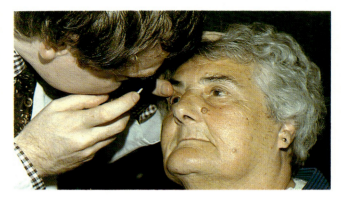

Fig.1.11   The position for using the direct ophthalmoscope.

Bruising of the retina shows up as a milky appearance of the normally transparent retina, while more severe damage will be accompanied by intraretinal and preretinal haemorrhage.

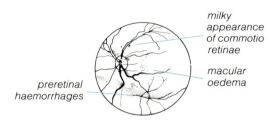

Fig.1.12   Severe contusion injury with retinal damage.

The underlying choroid may also be damaged, with semilunar splits that are often concentric with the optic disc; bleeding may occur underneath the retina.

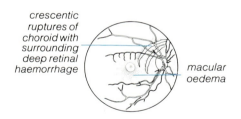

Fig.1.13   Choroidal ruptures after contusion.

Specialist techniques of examination

Slit-lamp microscopy
This technique is used to examine the anterior part of the eye in great detail: it gives an optical section of the eye by reflecting a fine beam of light obliquely into the eye, which is viewed through a powerful binocular microscope.

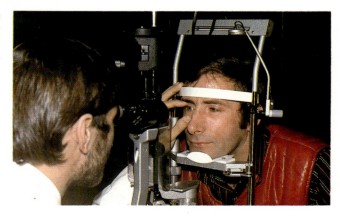

Fig.1.14   The binocular slit-lamp microscope in use.

The slit-lamp can be focused at varying depths from the cornea to the anterior vitreous, enabling anatomical relationships to be studied.

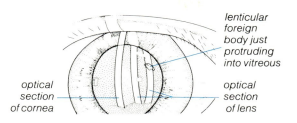

Fig.1.15 Slit-beam appearance of a foreign body in the lens protruding into the vitreous (slit-beam is from left).

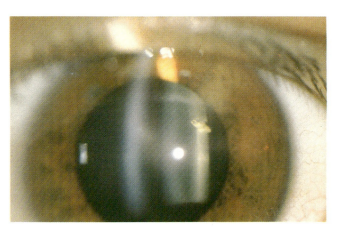

In closed eye injuries a three-mirror contact lens is used with the slit-lamp to examine parts of the eye inaccessible to the slit-beam alone; the mirrors are set at different angles to allow examination of the anterior chamber drainage angle, the peripheral and equatorial retina, while the central lens allows examination of the vitreous and posterior retina.

Another attachment to the slit-lamp allows measurement of intraocular pressure; this technique is known as applanation tonometry, as the pressure within the eye is measured against the force required to flatten a given surface area.

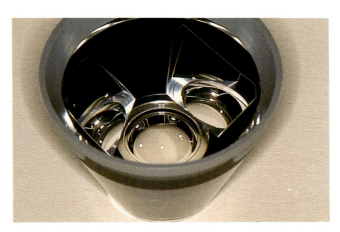

Fig.1.16 Three-mirror contact lens.

Indirect ophthalmoscopy

This technique of examining the fundus involves using a focused head-lamp and a condensing lens; it is particularly useful when the transparency of the media is impaired, as for example after a foreign body has traversed the lens of the eye.

The optics of the system allow examination of the peripheral retina and may reveal damage not readily visible with the direct ophthalmoscope. The low magnification allows large areas of the retina to be examined at any one time, and details of any abnormality can be mapped out for future reference.

Early assessment of the posterior segment after injury is very important, as later examination may be prevented by cataract formation or haemorrhage.

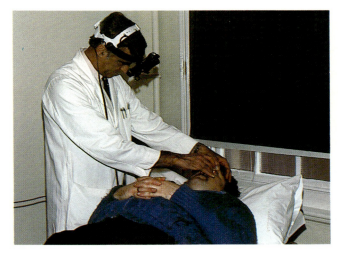

Fig.1.17 The indirect ophthalmoscope in use.

When to dilate the pupil

Pupil dilation is required for adequate examination of the lens and the structures behind it, and is therefore indicated in most injuries. 0.5% tropicamide drops are the first choice, since they are short-acting and reversible if required; if examination with the indirect ophthalmoscope or three-mirror contact lens is needed, 0.5% cyclopentolate and 10% phenylephrine drops are used.

The advantages of pupil dilation outweigh the small risk of precipitating further bleeding. In blunt injuries with blood in the anterior chamber, pupil dilation immobilises the damaged tissues and allows early examination of the posterior segment; only with tears involving the pupil margin should dilation be avoided.

Similarly with small perforating wounds, dilating the pupil can allow a better assessment of anterior segment damage which will be helpful during repair. Slit-lamp examination can distinguish between fibrin on the surface of the lens or damage to the lens itself.

Full dilation is mandatory when a posterior segment intraocular foreign body is suspected, as examination with the indirect ophthalmoscope will be required.

All the drops referred to are available as sterile single dose units.

Assessing an extraocular injury

Sometimes the brunt of the injury is borne by the tissues around the eye, so having excluded any major internal damage, the examination is completed by assessing any eyelid damage, testing eye movements and pupil reactions, and looking for signs of an orbital fracture.

Lid lacerations

Injuries such as windscreen accidents result in multiple facial lacerations and the eyelids are often involved. Typically the lacerations are deeply shelving from recoil onto the shattered glass, and an underlying ocular perforation is common if the eyelids are involved.

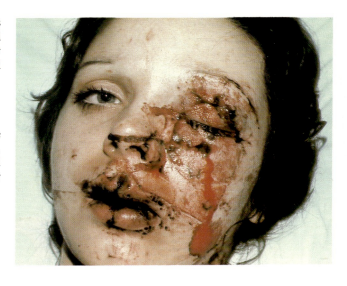

Fig.1.18 Facial lacerations after a windscreen injury.

Lacerations of the upper lid may damage the underlying levator muscle and orbital septum, and glass particles may be deeply embedded in the wound. If the laceration extends medially, the superior oblique tendon may be damaged as it passes through the trochlea leading to disabling torsional diplopia.

Any laceration that involves the eyelid margin will require careful repair to avoid notching, while those at the medial end should be examined to exclude damage to the lacrimal drainage system.

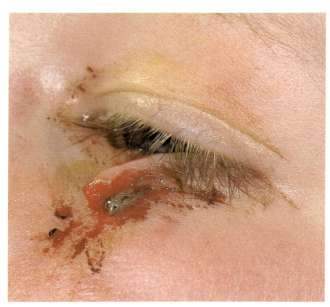

Fig.1.19 Torn lower canaliculus and lid laceration.

Ocular motility problems

Eye movements should be tested in all directions of gaze and the patient is asked whether there is any double vision. If eyelid swelling is present, the upper lid should be held up during the test, otherwise the defect may be missed; severe swelling may prevent full examination for a few days.

Misalignment of the globe can be assessed by noting the position of the corneal reflections from a torch light. Any protrusion or retraction of the globe is best observed from the side or from above.

Double vision following a blow on the eye may be a sign of an orbital fracture; this usually involves the orbital floor, and is known as a 'blow-out fracture'. It is accompanied by anaesthesia affecting the infraorbital nerve, and crepitus due to communication with an air sinus. Mechanical restriction of eye movements and enophthalmos result from herniation of soft tissues into the fracture line.

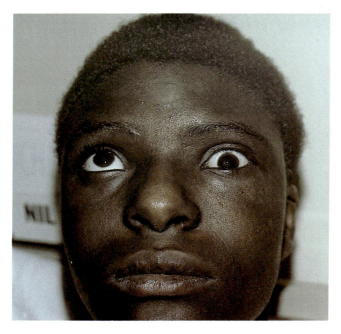

　Fig. 1.20 Restricted upgaze in a left blow-out fracture.

A blow to the eye may result in intraorbital haemorrhage with resulting proptosis and haemorrhagic swelling of the conjunctiva. In such an injury, damage to the structures at the apex of the orbit is common, resulting in optic nerve damage or a third nerve palsy. Initially the proptosis and tissue swelling make assessment difficult, and there is a risk of corneal and conjunctival exposure. In this type of injury internal ocular damage is common and an underlying rupture of the globe may also be present.

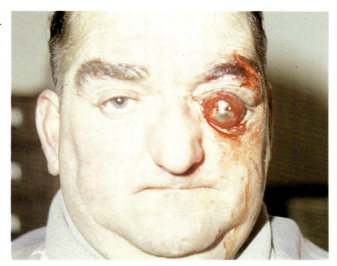

Fig.1.21 Haemorrhagic proptosis and a suspected posterior rupture of the globe from a severe blow to the orbit.

Pupil signs

An afferent pupil defect is a sign of optic nerve damage: the pupil fails to respond to direct light but constricts normally when the other eye is illuminated. This is a valuable sign in injuries such as optic nerve avulsion (see Fig.1.2), when vitreous haemorrhage obscures the view. If the optic nerve is damaged more posteriorly, the optic disc at first appears healthy but the vision is severely reduced; optic atrophy develops over the next few weeks.

An efferent pupil defect is unreactive to either direct or consensual stimulation; it may occur after a head injury and is a sign of raised intracranial pressure due to serious complications. When accompanied by ptosis and restricted eye movements, a third nerve palsy is present. Pupil involvement helps confirm the diagnosis in injuries associated with swelling and mechanical restriction of eye movements.

Care must be taken not to confuse an efferent pupil defect with traumatic mydriasis (a dilated pupil accompanying an hyphaema) or previous instillation of pupil-dilating drops.

Investigations

When to x-ray

All patients with a suspected intraocular foreign body must be x-rayed (particularly if a hammer has been used); it is the only reliable way of excluding this serious injury. For diagnostic purposes two P-A views and two lateral views of the orbit are taken in order to exclude artefacts. Particles from a hammer often have a characteristic semilunar shape.

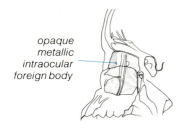

opaque
metallic
intraocular
foreign body

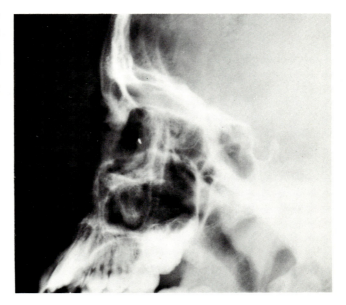

Fig.1.22 X-ray appearance of an intraocular foreign body.

Similarly all patients with an orbital injury must be x-rayed to exclude an underlying fracture, or where there is any question of a head injury.

At times it is difficult to decide whether to x-ray a patient with a perforating injury because of the risk of aggravating any damage. Certainly, if an extensive laceration is present it is better to limit the amount of manipulation involved; in this situation it may be preferable to use a portable x-ray machine to avoid moving the patient. If an x-ray is not taken preoperatively it should be performed subsequently in the postoperative period.

MINOR INJURIES: ABRASIONS AND LACERATIONS

This section will describe the presentation and treatment of minor abrasions and lacerations which can usually be dealt with in the Accident Department.

Corneal Abrasion

Typically this injury is caused by a finger-nail or a similar agent catching the eye; the condition is acutely painful, with a foreign body sensation in the eye and profuse watering.

Ciliary injection is present (capillary dilation around the limbus) and the loosened corneal epithelium has a translucent appearance. Epithelial loss can be confirmed by instilling a drop of 0.5% fluorescein which stains the denuded area bright green. A blue light enhances this appearance.

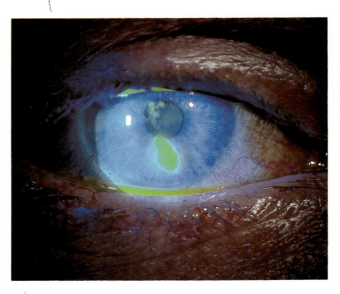

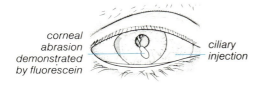

Fig.1.23 A corneal abrasion stained by fluorescein.

Treatment

The denuded surface of the cornea must be carefully inspected to exclude any foreign matter embedded in the surface; small particles of dirt may potentiate bacterial infection and will prevent perfect adhesion of the newly formed epithelium. This may lead to the syndrome of a recurrent corneal abrasion. If there is any foreign matter or a loose tag of epithelium, the surface should be gently wiped with a moist sterile cotton-wool bud, after anaesthetising the cornea with 0.4% benoxinate drops.

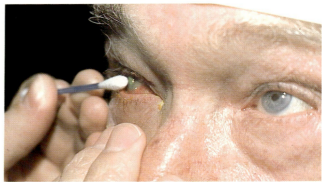

Fig.1.24 Debriding loose epithelium from a corneal abrasion.

The corneal epithelium heals by a rapid cell-slide to cover the defect and a slower multiplication of cells to restore the normal thickness. The surface is usually covered within 24 hours, but until this has occurred any lid movement will be painful.

0.5% chloramphenicol drops are instilled, and the eye is firmly padded for 24 hours. After this the eye can be uncovered, but the patient should be instructed to return if the pain has not improved.

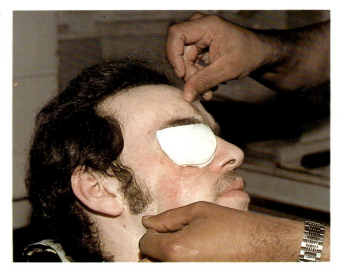

Fig.1.25 Firm eye pad applied.

Recurrent corneal abrasion

In some patients imperfect healing occurs, and for many months they periodically experience a recurrence of the foreign body sensation and watering; this generally occurs on waking when the eyes are first opened.

Treatment consists of repeating the debriding regimen and firm padding as initially, but also prescribing chloramphenicol ointment to be instilled liberally every night for several weeks to prevent the lid adhesion. The problem may remain troublesome for one or two years.

Superficial Conjunctival Laceration

A similar type of injury may cause a conjunctival laceration. It is less painful than a corneal abrasion, but bleeding occurs both on the surface and into the tissue plane beneath it; the laxity of the tissues allows blood to spread under the transparent conjunctiva on the surface of the globe, and the patient can be quite alarmed by the appearance.

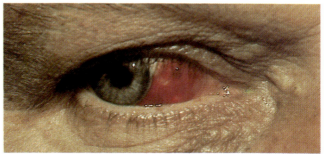

Fig.1.26 Conjunctival laceration with subconjunctival haemorrhage.

Treatment

The wound should be examined after instilling local anaesthetic drops; any surface blood and foreign particles are wiped away with a sterile cotton-wool bud. A small conjunctival laceration does not require suturing as it will heal rapidly without scarring, but if the underlying Tenon's capsule has been torn, suturing is required.

It is most important to exclude an underlying scleral perforation: if the subconjunctival haemorrhage is dense, preventing a view of the underlying sclera, the wound must be explored by opening up the subconjunctival tissues to expose the sclera and ensure there is no perforation. This is particularly important when the injury has been caused by a sharply pointed object, such as a dart. Prior to exploration, the pupil should be dilated for fundus examination to look for signs of internal damage from either contusion or perforation.

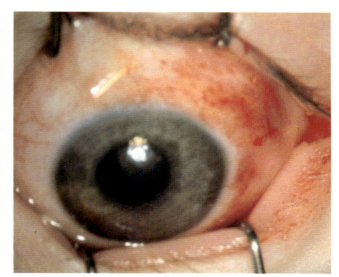

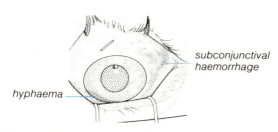

Fig.1.27 upper Subconjunctival haemorrhage from a dart injury.

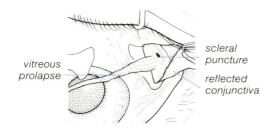

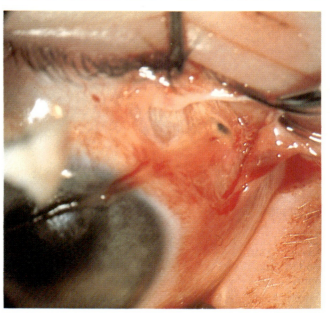

Fig.1.27 lower Exploration reveals a scleral perforation and vitreous prolapse.

If no scleral perforation is found, the conjunctiva is sutured using 0.7 metric (6/0) collagen, and antibiotic drops are prescribed four times a day for one week. The eye is padded overnight, but should be left uncovered from the next day.

If an underlying scleral perforation is present, this is a much more serious injury, and requires careful repair; this is discussed in Chapter 6.

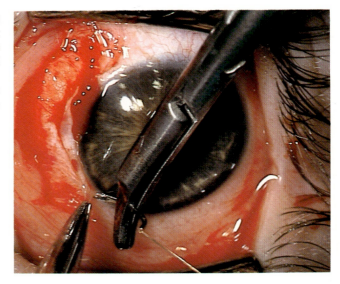

Fig.1.28 Suturing a conjunctival laceration.

Small Superficial Skin and Eyelid Lacerations

Small skin splits around the periorbital region are common after blunt injury to this region; there is often an associated haematoma. An underlying orbital fracture or contusion injury to the eye must be excluded.

Only small superficial skin splits or clean linear lacerations away from the eyelid tissues are suitable for repair in the Accident Department. More extensive lacerations, particularly those involving the eyelid margin or lacrimal drainage apparatus, should be cleaned and repaired in the main theatre under general anaesthesia.

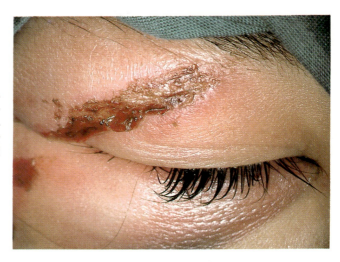

Fig.1.29 Split skin from a blow to the eye.

Treatment

Small linear skin splits lying in the natural skin folds can be taped with small butterfly dressings after carefully cleaning the wound. If they are perpendicular to the skin folds and tending to gape, suturing with 0.7 metric (6/0) polypropylene is required. Puncture wounds should be cleaned thoroughly and left unsutured.

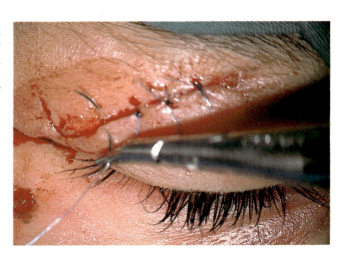

Fig.1.30 Ragged wound repaired with interrupted polypropylene sutures.

Longer skin lacerations that have not damaged the underlying muscle are repaired with an intradermal continuous suture using 0.7 metric (6/0) polypropylene, taking a bite of each dermal surface alternately and securing the two ends with doubled tape. The wounds are left uncovered and sutures are removed on the fourth or fifth day.

The treatment of more extensive lacerations and those involving the eyelid tissues is discussed in more detail in Chapter 2.

Glass Particles from Broken Spectacles

Spectacles with glass lenses can shatter on impact and result in multiple fine fragments of glass in the conjunctival sac; this causes an uncomfortable gritty feeling. Fragments often become trapped in the upper or lower fornices or under the plica medially. Sometimes fine slivers of glass become embedded in a partial thickness corneal laceration, and this will result in a sharp foreign body sensation. Occasionally the cornea is perforated.

Treatment

The first-aid treatment is to irrigate the conjunctival sac with sterile saline that has been warmed to body temperature. This should only be carried out if there is no obvious corneal perforation.

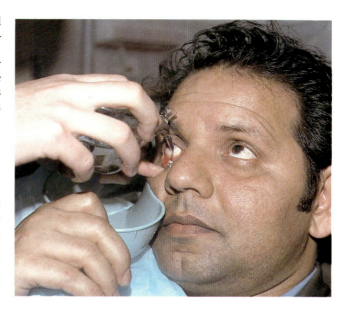

Fig.1.31   Irrigating the lower fornix.

The conjunctival fornices should be checked after this for any residual fragments; if present, the irrigation should be repeated. The cornea should then be stained with fluorescein, and examined on the slit-lamp for embedded particles.

In the absence of corneal damage, antibiotic drops are instilled and the eye is padded for a short period.

If corneal damage is present the eye will remain irritable for several days; antibiotic and atropine drops are instilled, and the eye is firmly padded. This treatment should be continued four times a day, and the patient should be reviewed to check for complications of infection or uveitis.

Glass Particles in the Cornea

Fine slivers of glass may have embedded in the superficial corneal stroma; if protruding, these can be removed on the slit-lamp using a fine needle. More deeply embedded particles under a shelving laceration may be less accessible to removal and if away from the axis of vision these are best left undisturbed.

If near the axis of vision, removal is performed under local anaesthesia using the magnification of the operating microscope; a fine needle can be used to manipulate the particles or they can be flushed out by irrigating with sterile saline via a fine canula (Rycroft).

If a deeply situated particle is projecting through to the anterior chamber, it may be safer to leave it alone if there is no aqueous leak; attempted removal may cause loss of the anterior chamber and damage to the lens. In this situation the patient should be admitted for a short period of observation and treated for a penetrating injury with systemic antibiotics.

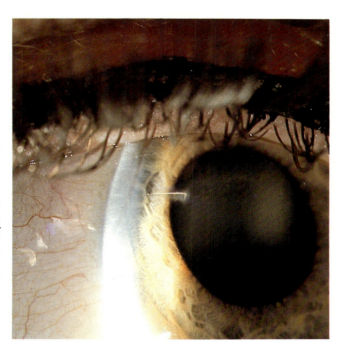

Fig.1.32 Deeply embedded glass particle projecting through the cornea.

Sometimes spontaneous inward migration of the particle occurs over a period of time, and it will eventually fall harmlessly to the bottom of the anterior chamber. It can be removed more safely from this position if it causes irritation.

If the wound is leaking around a particle or it is considered unsafe to leave, removal will need to be undertaken under general anaesthesia; similarly on occasions a large flap laceration of the cornea may need suturing even if there is no perforation. These techniques will be described in the chapter dealing with perforating injuries (see Chapter 6).

Many minor accidents occur in which bits of grit or splashes of liquid get into the eyes resulting in a superficial injury. This section will describe those which can be treated in the Accident Department, and how to recognise the more serious injuries requiring in-patient treatment.

Superficial Corneal Foreign Bodies (Metallic)

In an industrial area this is a common injury among people working on grinding machines: small steel particles fly off and hit the cornea, causing momentary discomfort. They have usually travelled with sufficient speed to embed on the surface of the cornea, but very occasionally such a foreign body can penetrate internally.

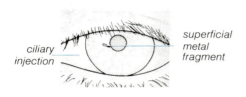
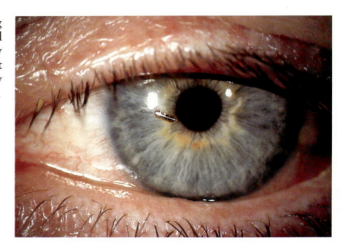

Fig.1.33 Fresh corneal foreign body.

If not examined and removed immediately, the particle starts to rust and the eye becomes inflamed and painful. The usual symptoms of corneal irritation develop within 12 to 24 hours with a foreign body sensation, photophobia and lacrimation. Dilation of the perilimbal vessels (ciliary injection) is present and may be localised to the limbus adjacent to the foreign body. The latter is visible as a small brown speck embedded on the corneal surface.

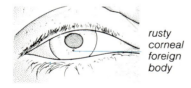
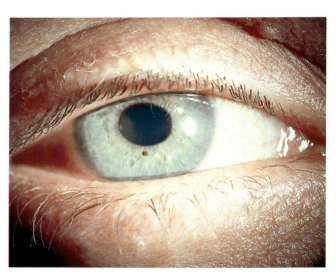

Fig.1.34 Brown discolouration of corneal foreign body.

If the foreign body has been present for a few days, a toxic reaction develops in the adjacent corneal stroma, leading to loss of transparency around the foreign body. Slit-lamp examination may show the presence of flare and cells in the anterior chamber, due to an associated inflammation of the iris and ciliary body (anterior uveitis).

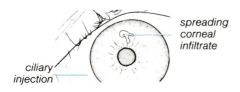
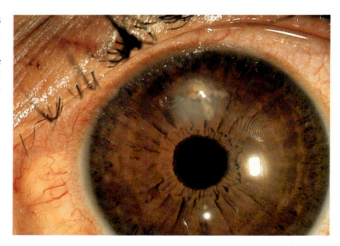

Fig.1.35 Toxic reaction to a corneal foreign body.

Secondary infection may develop, accompanied by worsening of the pain. This changes in character to a severe continuous ache accompanied by a drop in vision and a purulent discharge. A spreading infiltrate develops around the foreign body, and the anterior chamber becomes filled with exudate and cellular debris; this forms a white fluid level at the bottom of the anterior chamber (hypopyon), and is a sign of serious intraocular inflammation.

This complication can rapidly lead to panophthalmitis and destruction of the eye, and requires urgent treatment in hospital (see page 7.10).

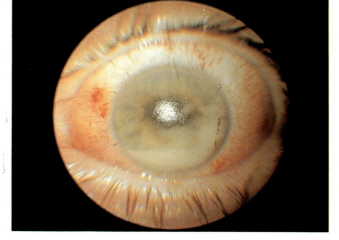

Fig.1.36 Infected corneal foreign body with hypopyon.

Treatment

The earlier the foreign body is removed the better, as this lessens the stromal reaction and ultimate scarring. The cornea is anaesthetised with benoxinate drops, and the foreign body can be prised off using a fine needle. The magnification of the slit-lamp microscope is helpful during this procedure.

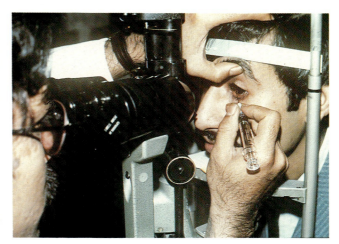

Fig.1.37 Removing a corneal foreign body with a sharp needle.

If the particle has been present for a few hours, a residual ring of rust remains. This may perpetuate inflammation and delay healing. It should be picked off with a needle as far as possible, or removed by using a battery-operated dental burr.

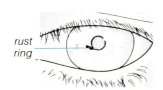

rust ring

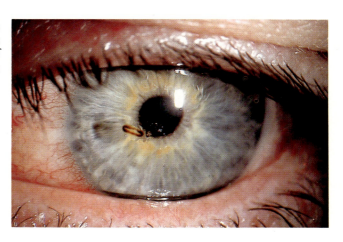

Fig.1.38 Residual rust after foreign body removal (cf. Fig.1.33).

Since the foreign body has damaged the corneal stroma, healing takes several days and may leave a persisting opacity.

Antibiotic drops are prescribed to prevent secondary infection, and 2% homatropine drops are given to relieve the pain from the associated uveitis. Epithelialisation of the defect will be slower than in a simple abrasion, and firm padding is required for a few days if rust has formed.

The patient should be instructed to return if there is any worsening of the pain. Patients with a stromal reaction from delayed removal should be seen in two days for reassessment.

CAUTION: Any patient with a history of using a hammer on steel must be examined in detail to look for a penetrating wound and signs of internal damage. An x-ray of the orbit is essential to exclude an intraocular foreign body.

Deep Corneal Foreign Bodies (Metallic)

Although the velocity of a fragment flying off a hammer is usually sufficient to penetrate the eye, occasionally these particles arrest in the deeper layers of the cornea. Their appearance is quite different from the superficial specks seen following a grinding or drilling injury. Hammer injuries have particles with a typical wedge or semilunar form.

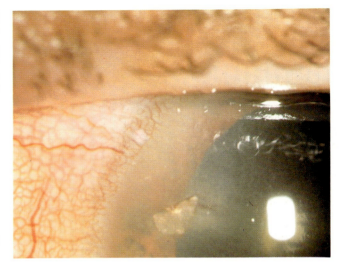

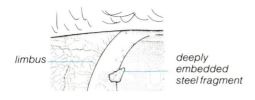

limbus

deeply
embedded
steel fragment

Fig.1.39 Hammering injury with a deep corneal foreign body.

These are more difficult to remove as they have usually travelled obliquely, and the tip may penetrate the anterior chamber.

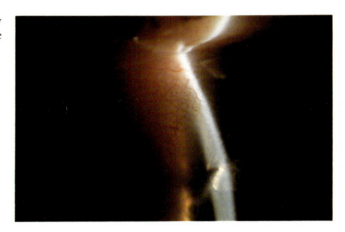

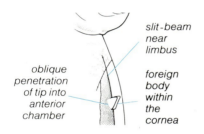

slit-beam
near
limbus

oblique
penetration
of tip into
anterior
chamber

foreign
body
within
the
cornea

Fig.1.40 Slit-beam showing deep penetration.

Treatment

Removal often necessitates slightly enlarging the corneal wound over the foreign body when it may be prised free with a needle or removed with a hand magnet. If the foreign body is known to be penetrating the anterior chamber, this should be performed in the Operating Theatre under general anaesthesia, as a corneal suture may be required to seal an aqueous leak. More superficial particles may be removed on the slit-lamp using a razor fragment and disposable needle.

Postoperatively these injuries have a mild uveitis and they need treatment with a topical antibiotic/steroid combination plus mydriatic drops for a few weeks.

Other Deep Corneal Foreign Bodies

Not all embedded corneal foreign bodies are from industrial injury; broken spectacles or windscreen accidents may result in glass particles embedded in the cornea (see Fig.1.32).

Pencil injuries are common in children, and in this example a fragment of an indelible pencil has resulted in staining of the corneal stroma.

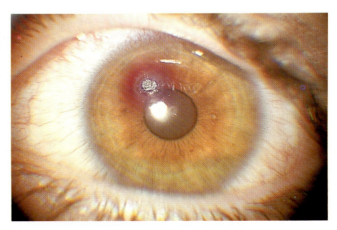

Fig.1.41 Indelible pencil injury with corneal staining.

Other Superficial Foreign Bodies

Airborne foreign bodies such as flies or smuts tend to get carried up into the upper fornix of the conjunctival sac by the reflex spasm of the lids and Bell's phenomenon (elevation of the eyes on forced lid closure). Soft objects will often be washed out by the reflex lacrimation, but particles of smut may embed on the inner surface of the upper lid and cause persistent irritation.

The patient presents with a foreign body sensation and a slightly injected eye; if no cause is found on the bulbar surface, the upper lid is everted over a wool bud or ointment applicator to examine the conjunctival surface: to do this the patient is instructed to keep looking down, and the upper lid is gently pulled downwards by traction on the eyelashes; the blunt applicator is then held against the upper margin of the tarsal plate, and the lid is everted over it. Eversion of the lid is corrected by instructing the patient to look up.

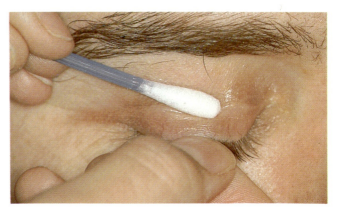

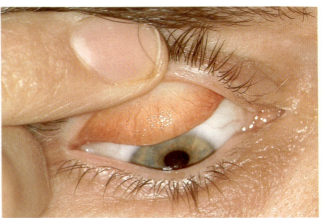

Fig. 1.42 upper & lower Everting the upper lid.

A subtarsal foreign body is often trapped in the sulcus behind the lid margin. It is usually a brown speck like a corneal foreign body.

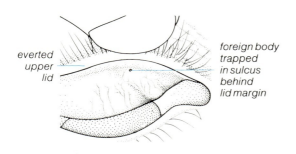

everted upper lid

foreign body trapped in sulcus behind lid margin

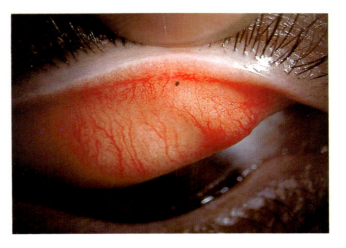

Fig.1.43 A subtarsal foreign body.

Instant relief is obtained by removing the foreign body using a moist cotton-wool bud.

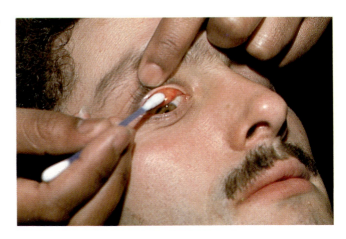

Fig.1.44 Removing a subtarsal foreign body.

1.17

Occasionally an embedded subtarsal foreign body may be neglected and become incorporated in a granuloma; the patient usually gives a history of a foreign body going in several weeks before, followed by discharge and swelling of the upper lid.

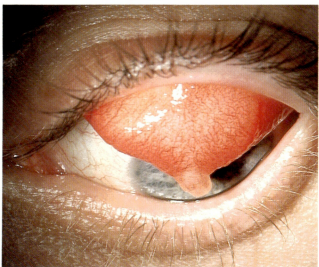

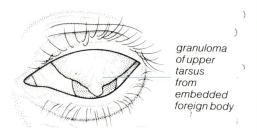

granuloma of upper tarsus from embedded foreign body

Fig.1.45   Upper lid granuloma due to an embedded brick particle.

The lesion requires incision and curettage from the tarsal surface, using a technique similar to that for a meibomian cyst. After infiltrating the skin with local anaesthetic and instilling amethocaine drops, the lid is everted with a meibomian clamp and the granuloma incised vertically. The foreign body may be encapsulated, requiring excision with scissors.

Hard contact lenses may also be trapped in this region causing similar granuloma formation; in this example the patient thought he had lost the lens several months before.

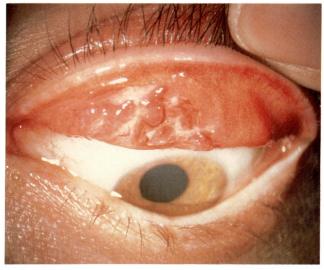

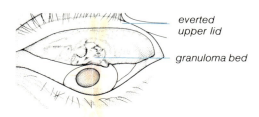

everted upper lid

granuloma bed

Fig.1.46   Granuloma bed after removal of a trapped contact lens.

A foreign body in this position may gradually erode into the lid and present as cystic lesion on the skin surface. This is removed via a horizontal incision in the eyelid skin, excising the cyst with scissors. In this example the cyst contained a lost contact lens.

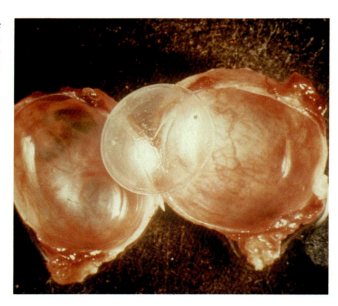

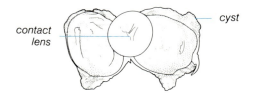

contact lens

cyst

Fig.1.47   Section of eyelid cyst containing a contact lens.

If there is no subtarsal foreign body, the superior fornix can be checked by lifting the everted upper lid with a glass rod after anaesthetising the surface with benoxinate drops. Flies and grass seeds trapped in this position may be removed by a glass rod covered with ointment; blunt forceps may sometimes be required.

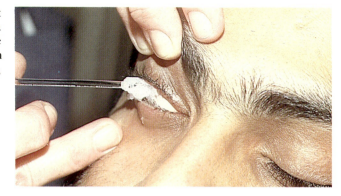

Fig.1.48 Checking the upper fornix with a glass rod.

The recess behind the plica may trap a foreign body; this should be examined with the eye abducted and the foreign body can be removed with a moist cotton-wool bud. An eyelash may sometimes impact in the punctum, with the broken end causing persisting irritation; fine forceps are used for removal.

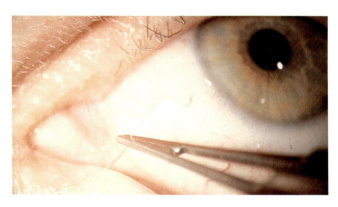

Fig.1.49 Removal of a broken eyelash from the punctum.

An uncommon superficial foreign body is the husk of a bird seed; the translucent dome-shaped husk acts like a suction cup and adheres to the conjuctiva or cornea. A similar effect may be produced by an insect wing-case. The suction effect makes it quite difficult to remove **unless** forceps are used.

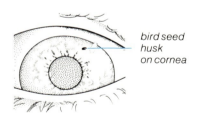

bird seed husk on cornea

Fig.1.50 Seed husk adhering to the cornea.

Contact lens wearers may present with a foreign body sensation in the eye; usually the symptoms have developed after wearing the lens for a longer period than usual. The vision blurs and the eyes become acutely painful and watery. Prolonged wear of a hard contact lens results in anoxia of the cornea, and leads to punctate staining of the epithelium.

Recovery occurs over 24 hours after which contact lens wear may be resumed; tolerance should be built up slowly if there has been a period of disuse.

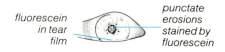

fluorescein in tear film   punctate erosions stained by fluorescein

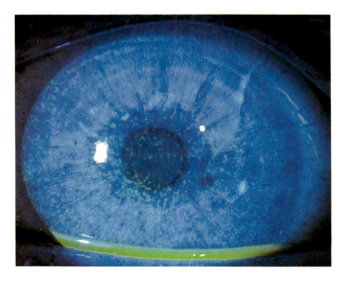

Fig.1.51 Corneal erosions after prolonged contact lens wear (illuminated with blue light).

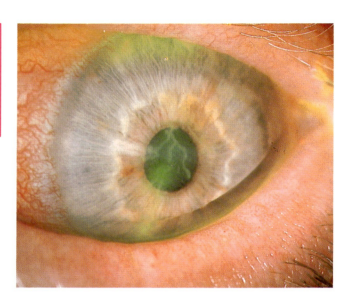

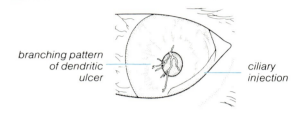

branching pattern of dendritic ulcer

ciliary injection

Fig.1.52 A dendritic ulcer of the cornea.

Minor Chemical Irritants and Burns

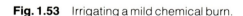

Household accidents with detergents, hot fat or paint are common; these are rarely serious unless a caustic substance such as liquid ammonia has been involved. Industrial accidents are often more serious, resulting from concentrated acid or caustic soda splashes, or from molten metal. A careful history should be taken to establish the exact nature of the burn and what treatment has been given.

The first-aid treatment is to irrigate the eye as soon as possible (at the scene of the accident, copious tap water should be applied immediately if sterile solutions are not to hand). Alkali burns penetrate deeply within seconds, and prolonged irrigation is required. This should be repeated in the Accident Department with sterile saline for at least half an hour.

In lime burns the fornices should be checked carefully for residual particles. These may need manual removal with forceps or a moist cotton-wool bud.

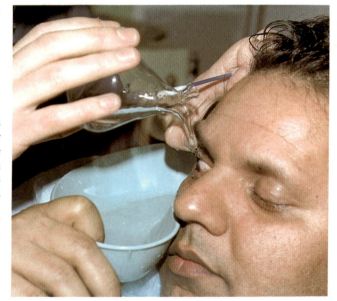

Fig. 1.53 Irrigating a mild chemical burn.

In mild burns the eyelids will be slightly red and swollen, and the conjunctival blood vessels will be hyperaemic. Fluorescein drops should be instilled to check for epithelial damage, and anything more than slight punctate staining should be regarded as a significant injury requiring admission to hospital.

For the less severe burns irrigation is performed and chloramphenicol ointment is instilled; the patient can be reassured that there is no serious injury.

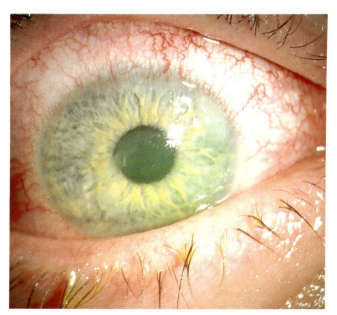

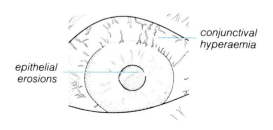

epithelial erosions

conjunctival hyperaemia

1.20   **Fig.1.54** Corneal damage from a splash of battery acid.

Molten metal will solidify on contact with the eye forming a cast, and the burn may involve the eyelids as well as the globe. The extent of damage depends on the temperature and volume of the molten metal. The cast will need removal with forceps after instilling benoxinate drops.

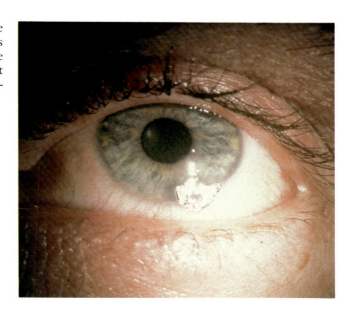

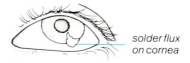
solder flux
on cornea

Fig.1.55 Mild corneal burn from solder flux.

With burns from molten metal at a very high temperature, the liquid flows into the lower fornix and over the lid margins causing serious injury. Localised necrosis occurs at the site of solidification.

Chemical burns from strong acids or alkalis cause widespread ocular damage; corneal clouding or ischaemia of the conjunctivae indicates a serious injury.

All patients with deep burns will need admission to hospital; their management is discussed in Chapter 4.

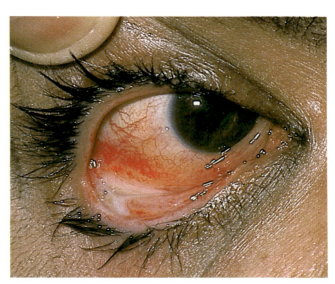

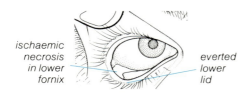
ischaemic
necrosis
in lower
fornix

everted
lower
lid

Fig.1.56 Ischaemia of the lower fornix from molten iron.

Burns from Ultraviolet Light

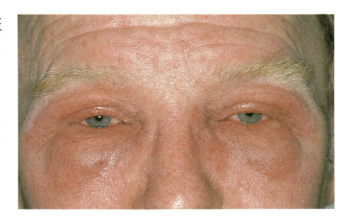

Welding flashes, incautious exposure to an ultraviolet lamp, or excessive sunlight (especially if reflected off white sand or snow) are the commonest causes of this problem.

Symptoms are not immediate because of the delayed effect of ultraviolet irradiation. The onset is usually about six hours after exposure, starting with a foreign body sensation in both eyes. This rapidly becomes increasingly severe accompanied by tense lid swelling and profuse lacrimation.

Fig.1.57 Burns from exposure to ultraviolet irradiation.

The corneal epithelium is damaged and shows widespread fine oedema, while the conjunctiva is hyperaemic and oedematous; in severe cases, fluorescein staining reveals punctate epithelial erosions. The condition is self-limiting but painful; local anaesthetic drops are first instilled, followed by an intensive regimen of anti-histamine drops. This is often ineffective when the condition has been present for some hours. Instillation of 0.5% prednisolone drops hourly, together with analgesic tablets and a double pad and bandage to close both eyes, will give some relief until healing occurs. In severe cases topical anaesthesia may need to be repeated.

1.21

Exploding Golf-Ball Injuries

An uncommon but problematical injury can occur in patients whose curiosity leads them to explore the inside of a golf-ball. If the external layers are penetrated, the semi-solid contents burst out under pressure and may squirt straight into the eyes. The exact nature of this substance is a trade secret, although it contains barium sulphate. The pultinaceous material may be forced under the conjunctiva via a small laceration, or may penetrate the eyelid skin, and a mild contusion injury of the globe may be present.

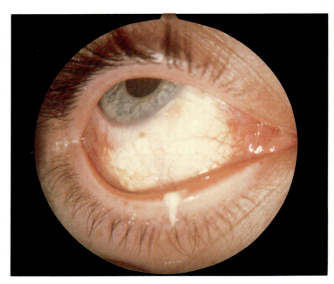

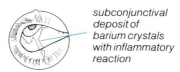

subconjunctival deposit of barium crystals with inflammatory reaction

Fig.1.58 Subconjunctival deposit from an exploding golf-ball. By courtesy of Professor W. Lee.

The substance is not acutely caustic but will lead to persisting irritation and granuloma formation if left under the conjunctiva. After instilling local anaesthetic drops, any surface material is wiped away with cotton-wool buds; subconjunctival deposits will need formal exploration and removal. 0.5% prednisolone drops are prescribed to reduce subsequent granuloma formation.

Histological studies after this type of injury have shown subconjunctival crystalline deposits with a surrounding inflammatory reaction. A granulomatous reaction develops with time.

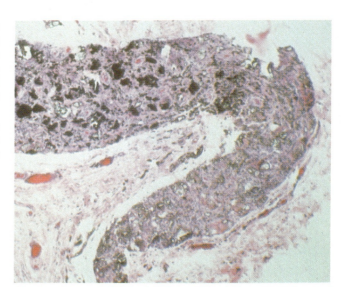

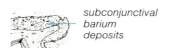

subconjunctival barium deposits

Fig.1.59 Histology 17 weeks after injury. By courtesy of Professor W. Lee.

Self-Inflicted Injuries

A chronic conjunctivitis that fails to respond to medical treatment may be self-induced; this should always be suspected when the lower fornix is exclusively affected, and when the appearance is atypical. Malingerers may instil substances like toothpaste into the lower fornix, causing a chronic conjunctivitis. In this example, a young girl has been instilling dried herbs in the mistaken belief this will make her eyes sparkle.

The advent of extremely powerful and almost instantaneous acrylic glues has occasionally led to an accident involving the eyes. The tube closely resembles that of eye ointment, and mistaken (or self-inflicted) instillation glues the lids together very firmly.

The glue is not toxic to the eye, but no attempt should be made to separate the eyelids; spontaneous separation occurs in about seven days without any harmful effect.

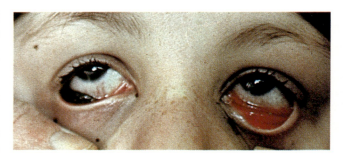

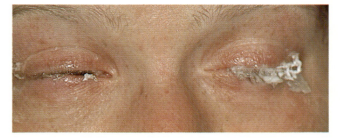

Fig.1.60 upper & lower Self-inflicted injuries: conjunctivitis artefacta and superglue instillation.

2

Lacerations of the Face, Eyelids and Lacrimal Drainage System

LACERATIONS OF THE FACE, EYELIDS AND LACRIMAL DRAINAGE SYSTEM

This chapter will discuss the general management of facial lacerations, particularly those that involve the eyelid tissues or the lacrimal drainage system.

Causes of Injury

Windscreen accidents often cause extensive facial and ocular injuries, but have become less common in the United Kingdom since the introduction of seat-belt legislation. In these injuries an underlying ocular perforation must be excluded. Bleeding coming from beneath the eyelids or a flattened appearance of the upper lid should suggest a serious ocular injury.

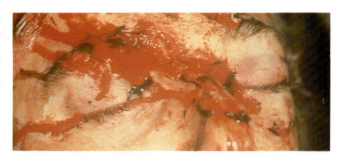

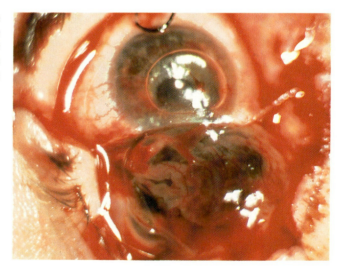

Fig. 2.1 upper Windscreen injury with extensive facial lacerations. Note flattening of both upper lids and bleeding from the right eye.
Fig. 2.1 lower Underlying bilateral perforating eye injuries. By courtesy of Mr. H.K. Mehta.

Assault or accidents with knives or broken glass have become the commonest causes of lacerations around the eye, often with serious damage to the globe. These injuries may have deep puncture wounds, and the eye should be carefully examined for a posterior perforating wound.

Fig. 2.2 Lid laceration from stab wound with scleral perforation and retinal prolapse.

A small number of injuries are caused by animal bites, which result in ragged wounds with crushed tissues; they may involve tissue loss and have a higher risk of infection.

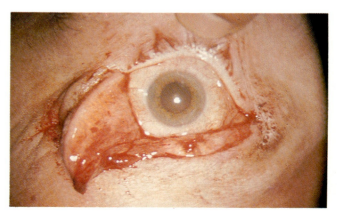

2.2   **Fig. 2.3** Eyelid injury from a dog bite.

A preliminary assessment of these injuries will have been carried out in the Accident Department. The initial management includes taking a history and conducting the examination as outlined earlier; it is important to achieve temporary haemostasis to any major bleeding vessel. Antibiotic and tetanus cover should be given (see page 1.3).

In the past, immediate repair of lacerations was advised, because of the risk of infection and tetanus; however, with careful surgical toilet, modern antibiotics and immunisation against tetanus, the risk of these complications is now much less, and it is preferable to delay surgery a few hours until optimal conditions are available. Complex facial and lid lacerations are best repaired under general anaesthesia, as this allows adequate surgical toilet and full assessment of the extent of the injuries.

FACIAL LACERATIONS

General Principles of Repair

1. *Thorough cleansing of all wounds* should precede any attempt at repair; this involves removal of all foreign matter such as glass fragments from a shattered windscreen.

Wounds with embedded grit should be thoroughly cleaned, using a stiff brush to remove the dirt; failure to do this results in tattooing. Animal bites should be cleansed with an antiseptic solution, and puncture wounds should be left open as infection is likely.

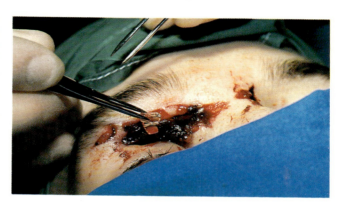

Fig. 2.4 Windscreen glass being removed from a deep laceration.

2. Wherever possible, *conservation of tissues* should be the aim: the blood supply to the face and eyelid region is so adequate that large flaps of skin have a good chance of surviving even if they appear devitalised.

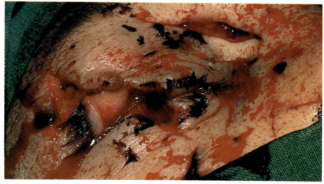

Fig. 2.5 Complex eyelid laceration showing impaired perfusion.

As soon as haemostasis and tissue apposition are achieved, skin perfusion improves.

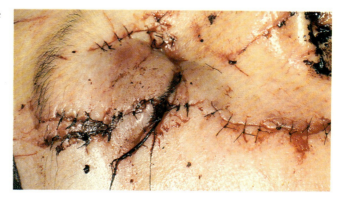

Fig. 2.6 Rapid improvement in skin colour by the end of repair.

3. The principle of conservation is extended to *tissue loss* in injuries such as a dog bite, where a piece of skin may have been bitten off; if still available and washed clean in antiseptic solution, the tissue is replaced as a free graft. Otherwise major tissue loss should be repaired by grafting or rotating a flap of similar tissue.

4. *A meticulous repair* of all layers of damaged tissues should be carried out.

If the laceration is running across the muscle fibres or penetrates deeply to involve periosteum, it will require careful suturing of the two layers, using interrupted deep and superficial stitches. Lacerations parallel with the muscle fibres will not need suturing of this layer.

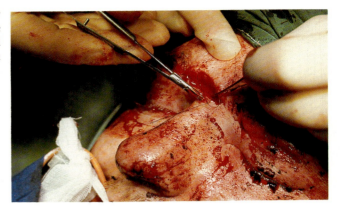

Fig. 2.7 A laceration of the forehead requiring deep sutures.

Repair of the muscle layer is followed by closure of the dermal tissues, using mattress sutures placed intradermally parallel to the wound to allow skin closure that is not under any tension. If this is not done, stretching of a scar that is running against the natural skin folds leads to an unsightly appearance.

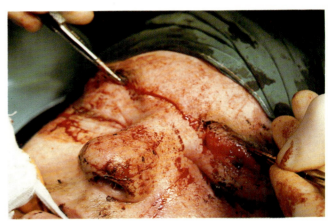

Fig. 2.8 Intradermal sutures achieving good skin approximation.

Skin closure is then completed using skin hooks to avoid any additional tissue damage from the use of forceps.

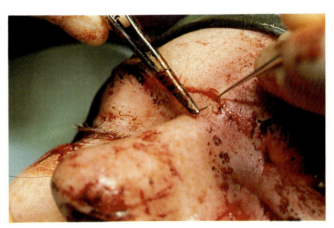

Fig. 2.9 Skin closure using skin hooks.

The deeper tissues can be repaired with 1 metric (5/0) collagen or polyglactin, while the skin is repaired with 0.7 metric (6/0) polypropylene. Skin sutures are removed on the third or fourth day after repair. Multiple lacerations will be accompanied by local oedema which improves as healing takes place.

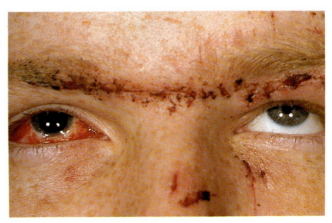

2.4   **Fig. 2.10** Facial lacerations one week after repair.

LACERATIONS INVOLVING THE EYELID STRUCTURES

Full-thickness Lid Lacerations Involving the Lid Margin

These lacerations transect the structures of the eyelid, cutting the lid margin, the tarsal plate and conjunctiva, orbicularis fibres, and the finer skin of the eyelid region.

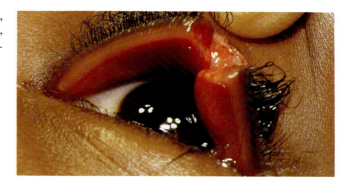

Fig. 2.11 Lid laceration splitting the tarsal plate.

As these lacerations run across the natural skin folds, careful cleaning of all foreign material and meticulous repair in layers is very important, otherwise contracture of the scar will lead to deformities of the lid margin. Those involving the lower lid may lead to ectropion with chronic watering of the eye and an unsightly appearance. Contracture of the scar in an upper lid laceration is more serious, as it leads to corneal exposure; this causes considerable discomfort and there is a risk of complications leading to loss of vision.

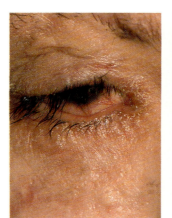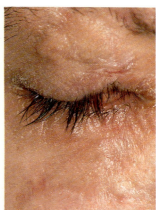

Fig.2.12 left Cicatrisation of eyelid scars resulting in exposure keratitis.
Fig. 2.12 right Upper lid contracture preventing closure.

After thorough cleaning, the laceration is inspected under magnification to identify damaged tissues and to plan repair; operating telescopes are the most suitable for this, giving low magnification and a wide field of vision. The operating microscope may also be used.

Eyelid tissues are delicate and the instruments used in the surgical repair should be as fine as those used in intraocular surgery. The eyelid margin is difficult to hold in forceps, and crushing or tearing of the lid margin will occur if coarse instruments are used.

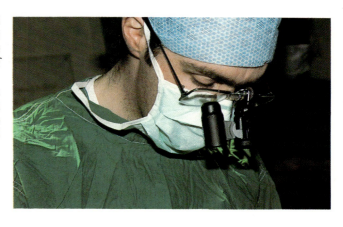

Fig. 2.13 Operating telescopes for repair of lid lacerations.

Time should be spent identifying anatomical landmarks particularly in shelving wounds or those involving the medial canthus, as alignment may be difficult in these situations. If care is not taken over this, alignment may be faulty, and the lash margin may be deviated into the wound. In complex lacerations, particularly those running obliquely and shelving, a lid margin suture is placed first, and the alignment of tissues is tested. It may then be necessary to place the tarsal sutures before tying the lid margin suture.

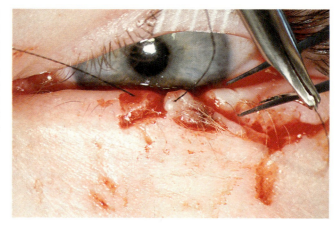

Fig. 2.14 Aligning the lid margin in a complex laceration.

In vertical lacerations it is easiest to repair the tarsal plate first. The repair is performed by taking half-thickness bites, placed so that the knots lie on the skin side of the wound. Interrupted sutures are easier to align correctly compared with a continuous one, and should be placed at the apex of the wound first. Traditionally 0.7 metric (6/0) collagen or nylon have been the sutures of choice but newer materials such as 0.7 metric (6/0) polyglactin handle much better and make the surgery easier.

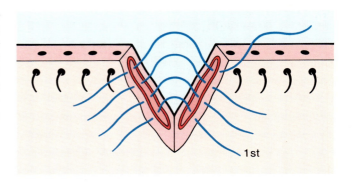

Fig. 2.15 Repairing the tarsal plate.

The eyelid margin should be reconstituted with a suture through the grey line (between the eyelashes and the meibomian gland orifices); 0.5 metric (7/0) silk is used rather than nylon, as the latter forms a stiff knot that may cause corneal irritation. The lips of the wound are slightly everted during suturing to ensure good coaptation; the margin should appear slightly heaped-up when the suture is tied. A further suture is placed just behind this, and one just in front; this three-suture technique reduces the incidence of lid notching. The suture ends are left long so they can be taped away from the margin at the end of the repair; they can also provide useful traction during repair.

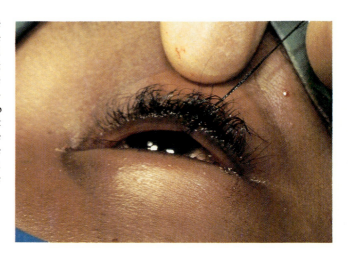

Fig. 2.16 Triple suture repair of lid margin

A vertical laceration will have cut across the fibres of the orbicularis but will be parallel to the levator muscle in the upper lid; oblique lacerations will cut across both. Transected muscle fibres should be repaired using 0.5 metric (7/0) polypropylene or 0.7 metric (6/0) polyglactin sutures. Skin closure is completed with interrupted 0.5 metric polypropylene or silk sutures.

Skin wounds are left dry and uncovered, but antibiotic ointment is instilled regularly into the conjunctival sac. Skin sutures are removed on the third or fourth day, leaving the marginal sutures until ten days. Clean lacerations usually heal well, resulting in normal lid function.

Avulsion of the Lower Eyelid

This injury is caused by an object 'hooking' the lower eyelid and tearing it from the medial canthus; bicycle-handle accidents or a dog bite may cause this. The inferior canaliculus is torn, disrupting the lower attachment of the medial ligament.

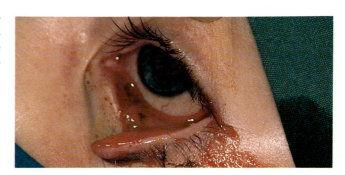

Fig. 2.17 Avulsion of the lower eyelid and medial ligament.

These injuries have shelving irregular wounds, and great care must be taken to align tissues correctly. Failure to do this results in ectropion of the lower lid, leading to a watery eye from eversion of the punctum and failure of the lacrimal pump mechanism. The surgical management is discussed in the section on damage to the lacrimal drainage apparatus (page 2.10).

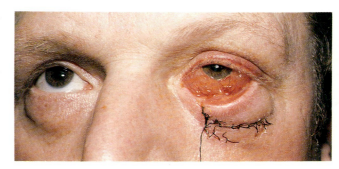

Fig. 2.18 Ectropion from failure to align tissues correctly.

Damage to the levator tendon

Deep lacerations running across the upper eyelid are common after a windscreen injury, and damage to the levator aponeurosis is likely. Medially the laceration may extend across the bridge of the nose and be continuous with a laceration on the other side. Lateral extension may damage the lacrimal gland, with a risk of subsequent fistula formation. Rarely a 'hook' injury of the upper lid may occur, splitting the levator aponeurosis through a small lid laceration.

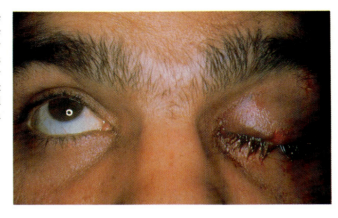

Fig. 2.19 Hook injury to the upper lid severing the levator muscle. By courtesy of Mr. D. Common.

Repair requires identification of the severed levator aponeurosis; it is useful to inspect the wound prior to anaesthesia, as attempted lid movement may help identify strands of the levator muscle. In some cases it is best to perform the repair under local anaesthesia, so as to confirm the levator fibres during surgery. If the levator muscle can be identified, it should be reattached to the distal portion or to the upper border of the tarsal plate (for suture material see page 2.6).

Postoperatively, lid oedema makes assessment difficult. Dimpling of the skin on either side of the upper lid on upgaze indicates some levator function and good recovery can usually be expected.

Failure to remove foreign material will leave a chronic granuloma and persisting ptosis; splinters of wood are the commonest cause of this problem.

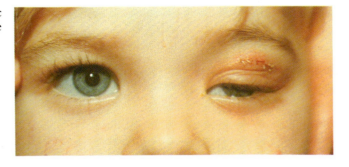

Fig. 2.20 Mechanical ptosis from a retained foreign body. By courtesy of Mr. H.K. Mehta.

The wound should be explored and any foreign material removed.

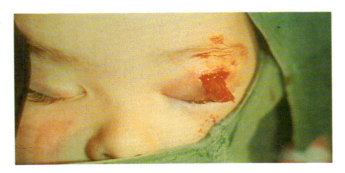

Fig. 2.21 Wood fragment found embedded in the wound. By courtesy of Mr. H.K. Mehta.

After thorough cleaning, repair is carried out as described above.

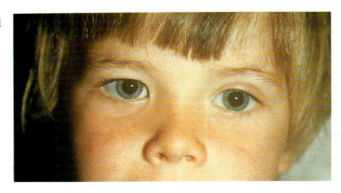

Fig. 2.22 Improvement of ptosis after secondary repair. By courtesy of Mr. H.K. Mehta.

Damage to the orbital septum

Higher lacerations dividing the orbital septum lead to herniation of fat into the wound.

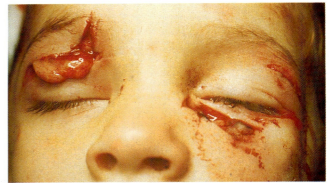

Fig. 2.23 Deep laceration of the upper lid with herniation of fat. By courtesy of Mr. S.S.F. Munro.

These injuries usually result from shattered glass and multiple particles may be embedded in the tissues; preoperative x-rays may help demonstrate this.

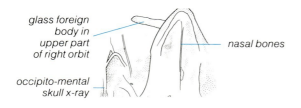

glass foreign body in upper part of right orbit

nasal bones

occipito-mental skull x-ray

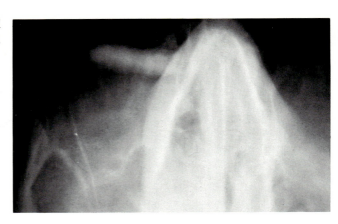

Fig. 2.24 Windscreen glass visible on x-ray.

The wound should be gently probed with a blunt instrument to identify foreign particles and to assess the depth of the wound. Thorough cleaning and removal of any foreign material is carried out and haemostasis is achieved; damage to the ethmoidal vessels may cause troublesome bleeding, and suction is needed to obtain an adequate view to clamp and tie the bleeding point. The orbital septum is repaired with 0.7 metric (6/0) collagen or polyglactin, and the overlying orbicularis and skin lacerations are repaired as described earlier.

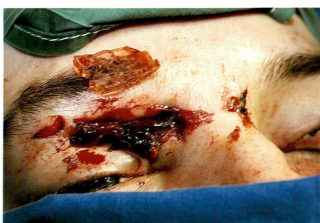

Fig. 2.25 Large glass fragment removed during repair.

These injuries may also damage the superior oblique tendon as it passes through the trochlea, or the trochlea itself may be detached; if identified, this should be reattached to the periosteum with 0.7 metric (6/0) nylon. However in most cases gross contusion of tissues makes identification and repair difficult.

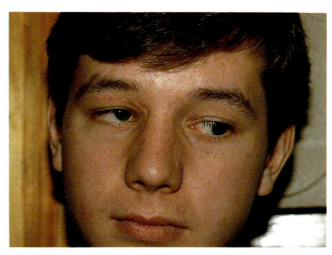

Fig. 2.26 Superior oblique palsy from the above injury.

Lid Lacerations Involving Tissue Loss

Full-thickness loss of eyelid tissues is fortunately a rare injury; more commonly partial thickness loss of skin and muscle occurs. Full-thickness skin grafts or flaps are applied to avoid subsequent contracture and distortion of the eyelid margin. The edges of the defect are made perpendicular, to facilitate apposition of the graft margin.

Total loss of eyelid tissues exceeding a quarter of the width will require reconstruction. Less than this amount can be repaired directly after squaring the edges; this applies both to the upper and lower eyelids, as there is sufficient laxity in the tissues to allow direct repair.

Extensive loss of the upper lid needs urgent repair, otherwise corneal exposure will occur. The defect can be improved by techniques using tissue from the lower lid, reconstructing the latter with a free mucosal and full-thickness skin graft or rotation flap if more than half of the lower lid has been used. This latter procedure is also used for lower lid defects.

These techniques are described in more detail in texts on ophthalmic plastic surgery and will not be discussed further here.

Early complications after repair of facial and eyelid lacerations

If an inexpert repair has been carried out and misalignment of the tissues is recognised within 36 hours of injury, it is possible to undo the initial repair and reconstitute the anatomical relationships. After this early period, it is better to defer any reconstructive surgery for at least six months, until the scars become less hypertrophic.

Occasionally severe tethering and shortening of an upper lid laceration from faulty primary repair leads to corneal exposure with a risk of ulceration and loss of the eye. Generally this results from failure to clean the wound adequately, so that retained foreign material stimulates fibrosis. In this situation early intervention is required, with excision of the scar and foreign material, followed by a further repair.

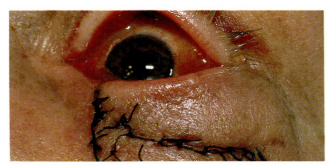
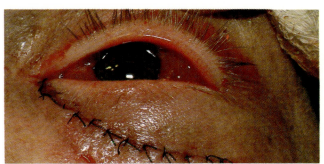

Fig.2.27 upper Ectropion from failure to align tissues correctly (see also Fig. 2.18).
Fig.2.27 lower Early secondary repair to improve alignment.

Lacerations involving the Lacrimal Drainage System

Tear drainage depends on correct positioning of the tear puncta in relation to the lacus of tears, proper functioning of the lacrimal pump system controlled by the medial ligament and the orbicularis muscle, and patency of the tear drainage system. Factors influencing eyelid position have already been discussed; this section will discuss the management of direct damage to the lacrimal passages.

The commonest site of damage is the lower canaliculus; less commonly the upper canaliculus is cut, or both may be involved. Infrequently the laceration is more medial, damaging the common canaliculus or lacrimal sac.

Long-term reviews have emphasised that one intact canaliculus can cope with basal lacrimal secretions, and that symptoms are minimal. Attempts to intubate both canaliculi when only one is disrupted carries the risk of damaging the common canaliculus; instruments such as the pigtail probe for introducing nylon thread or silicone tubes are to be avoided, as anatomical intubation is rarely achieved and false passages result from its use. It is doubtful whether direct suturing or temporary intubation of one canaliculus has any advantage over a simple lid repair, but these techniques help in alignment of tissues during repair.

Management of lacerations of the punctum or individual canaliculi

A laceration that runs through the punctum or very close to it can be managed by simple apposition of the eyelid tissues as described earlier, accompanied by a 3-snip operation to externalise the canaliculus onto the conjunctival surface proximal to the scar.

Where one canaliculus is damaged, the cut ends can be identified under the operating microscope; the proximal end is best visualised by injecting a small amount of diluted methylene blue dye via the intact canaliculus. This helps to identify anatomical landmarks during repair, so that an accurate alignment can be carried out.

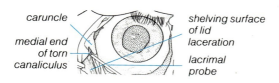

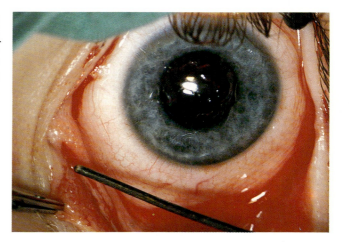

Fig. 2.28 Identifying the medial end of a lacerated canaliculus.

It is important to suture the inner aspect of the wound first, as exposure in this confined area is very difficult.

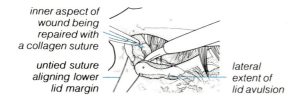

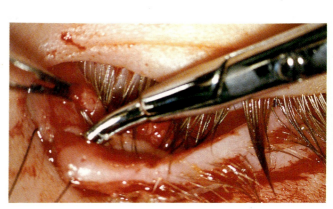

Fig. 2.29 Aligning the inner aspect of the laceration.

The cut ends of the severed canaliculus can be directly sutured at one point using 0.4 metric (9/0) polyamide, or a silicone tube may be threaded into the sac to splint the tissues during the rest of the repair. At the end of the procedure the silicone tube can be strapped to the forehead; it is usually lost within a couple of days.

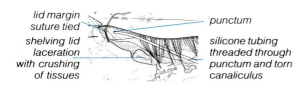

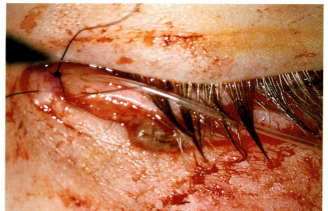

Fig. 2.30 Splinting the lower canaliculus during eyelid repair.

In lacerations transecting both canaliculi intubation is essential. In an adult it may be possible to achieve this through the nasolacrimal duct using silicone tubing attached to a flexible introducer; the ends of the probes are identified in the nose using a nasal speculum and head-light, and are brought out through the nostril and secured together. If direct intubation is not possible, a dacryocystorrhinostomy should be performed, otherwise a persistently watery eye will result. The silicone tubing is left in situ for twelve months.

Management of lacerations involving the common canaliculus or sac

Lacerations involving the common canaliculus or lacrimal sac are fortunately rare; when present they are often part of an extensive injury often involving tissue loss, disinsertion of the medial ligament and underlying fractures. In this situation it is best to concentrate on restoring the anatomy of the medial ligament and canthal tissues by transnasal wiring. If the damaged sac can be identified, intubation through the nasolacrimal duct can be attempted or if conditions are suitable, a dacryocystorrhinostomy with intubation should be performed. In practice, conditions are rarely favourable and secondary reconstruction may be required after several months (see naso-orbital fractures, page 3.9, and late reconstruction, page 10.5).

3
Orbital Injuries

FRACTURES OF THE ORBIT

This chapter will describe the presentation and management of fractures involving the orbit, and soft tissue injuries to the periocular structures and optic nerve. The ophthalmic complications of head and other injuries will be briefly described.

Fractures Involving the Inferior Orbital Wall

Infraorbital rim

The familiar 'black eye' arises from a diffuse blow to the orbit, which leads to bruising and oedema of the eyelids. The blow may be sufficient to cause a fracture of the infraorbital rim at the point where it is weakened by the canal for the infraorbital nerve; contusion of the nerve results in anaesthesia affecting the cheek.

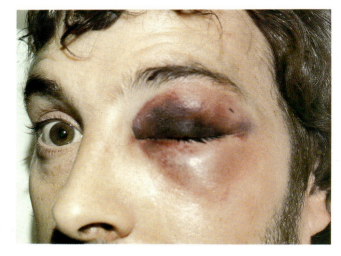

Fig. 3.1 'Black eye' from a fracture of the left infraorbital rim.

The fracture is confirmed by an occipito-mental x-ray which outlines the infraorbital rim. Ocular damage is uncommon, and motility is not disturbed unless there is an associated compression fracture of the orbital floor (vide infra); no specific treatment for isolated rim fractures is required.

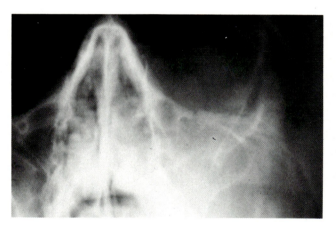

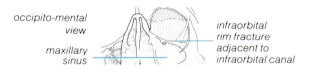

occipito-mental view

maxillary sinus

infraorbital rim fracture adjacent to infraorbital canal

Fig. 3.2 X-ray demonstrating a fracture of the left infraorbital rim.

Orbital floor

A blow to the infraorbital rim may result in a compression fracture extending into the orbital floor, or the force may be transmitted via the globe resulting in a classical 'blow-out fracture'.

Typically such an injury is caused by the impact of a rounded object slightly larger than the orbital margin; displacement of the globe posteriorly transmits the force to the orbital walls which give way at their weakest point. Blow-out fractures most commonly affect the posteromedial part of the orbital floor; the medial wall may also be affected, and rarely the roof.

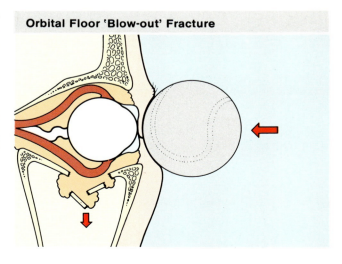

Orbital Floor 'Blow-out' Fracture

Fig. 3.3 Diagram illustrating the mechanism of a blow-out fracture.

Presentation

The patient presents with bruising and oedema of the eyelids. If seen within a few hours of injury, surgical emphysema with crepitus is often present; this is because air has entered the periorbital tissues via a fracture into the maxillary or ethmoid sinus. Often this is exacerbated when the patient sneezes or blows his nose, causing considerable alarm.

Anaesthesia in the distribution of the infraorbital nerve is common, with impairment or loss of sensation affecting the medial aspect of the cheek, the side of the nose and the medial part of the upper lip.

The other clinical features of a blow-out fracture may be masked in the early stages by lid oedema; the patient may not present for a few days until the swelling subsides, when he becomes aware of double vision as the eyelids start to open. The commonest restriction of eye movement is up and out, from entrapment of the inferior rectus muscle or adjacent connective tissue. The inferior oblique muscle may also be involved. The degree of limitation may range from minimal restriction of extreme upward gaze to no movement above the midline.

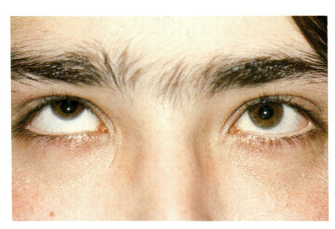

Fig.3.4 Restriction of left elevation after a blow-out fracture.

Less commonly, downgaze is affected, either alone or in combination with restriction of upgaze. In this situation the tethering of the globe is more marked, and there is often a manifest vertical deviation of the affected eye in the primary position of gaze. Double vision will be present in almost all positions of gaze.

Whether up or down movement is affected may depend on the position of the eye at the moment of impact and the degree of incarceration; it is claimed that the type of restriction helps predict the position of the fracture, but this is not reliable.

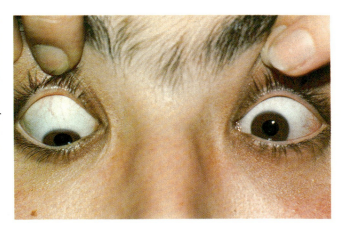

Fig.3.5 Restricted left depression after a blow-out fracture.

Enophthalmos is difficult to detect in the early stages if marked lid swelling and oedema of the orbital tissues are present; once this begins to subside, careful measurements with an exophthalmometer will confirm any enophthalmos. Clinically, the disparity between the two eyes may be apparent when viewed from below. Enophthalmos may be minimal in the primary position, but marked retraction of the globe may be present on attempted up- or downgaze if these movements are restricted. This is best observed from the side.

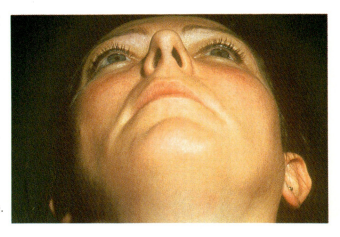

Fig.3.6 Enophthalmos of the left eye after a blow-out fracture. By courtesy of Mr. M.J.C. Wake.

Forced duction test

The test confirms entrapment of tissues and may occasionally help to release them; it involves determining the passive range of eye movement. The conjunctiva is anaesthetised with benoxinate drops and grasped near the limbus with blunt forceps; the patient is instructed to look in the restricted direction and the movement is assisted mechanically. Assessing mild degrees of limitation is difficult and it may be helpful to compare the range of the injured eye with the healthy one.

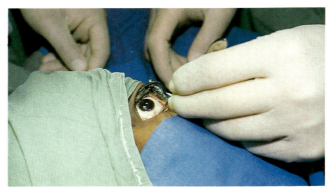

Fig.3.7 upper Forced duction test: elevation restricted prior to surgery.

This procedure should also be carried out at the start of a surgical exploration to identify entrapment of tissues, and should be repeated at the conclusion of surgery to confirm free movement.

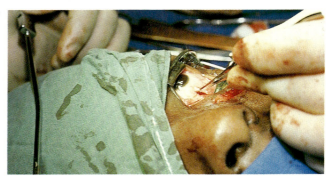

Fig.3.7 lower Full elevation at the end of surgery.

Radiological examination

Routine sinus views may show an opacity in the maxillary sinus from bleeding into this cavity. Air may also be visible in the periorbital tissues.

The orbital floor is best seen in a 15° up-tilt occipitomental view. Depressed bony fragments may be visible, and a 'hanging drop' from herniation of orbital tissues into the maxillary sinus is characteristic.

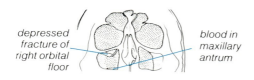

depressed fracture of right orbital floor

blood in maxillary antrum

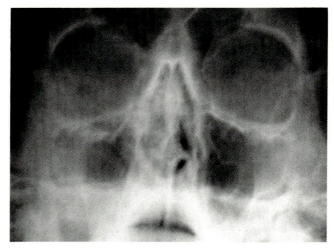

Fig. 3.8 Depressed 'trap-door' fracture of the right orbital floor.

Tomograms will help locate the position and extent of the fracture, but as this investigation involves quite a lot of radiation, this should only be considered in patients requiring surgical intervention.

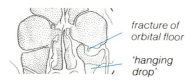

fracture of orbital floor

'hanging drop'

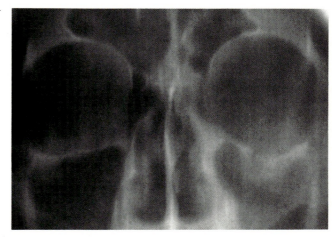

Fig. 3.9 Tomogram showing left posteromedial blow-out fracture with herniation of orbital tissues ('hanging drop'). By courtesy of Mr. M.J.C. Wake.

Improvement in computerised tomography techniques has allowed better definition of the orbit both in axial and coronal views; these techniques demonstrate soft tissue structures as well as bone and can, on occasions, confirm entrapment of the inferior rectus muscle.

Other damage may be demonstrated, such as a subperiosteal haematoma, and this is particularly helpful in the management of fractures complicated by retrobulbar haemorrhage (see Fig.3.42).

Early management of blow-out fractures

Minimal involvement with little or no restriction of eye movement is quite common; patients should be advised not to blow their nose forcefully, otherwise air may be forced into the orbital tissues. All patients should receive a course of antibiotics, to prevent infection spreading from the paranasal sinuses; orbital cellulitis may otherwise develop.

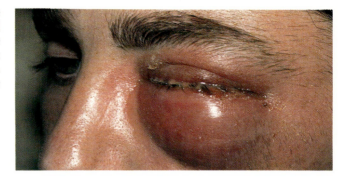

Fig. 3.10 Orbital cellulitis complicating a blow-out fracture.

Patients with significant restriction of eye movements should be admitted to hospital for observation, and a full orthoptic assessment should be carried out. The Hess test or Lee screen provides a measure of the restriction which can be repeated daily to monitor progress. The typical appearance of the chart for a blow-out fracture shows a compressed box for the affected eye (c.f. clinical appearance, Figs.3.4 and 3.5).

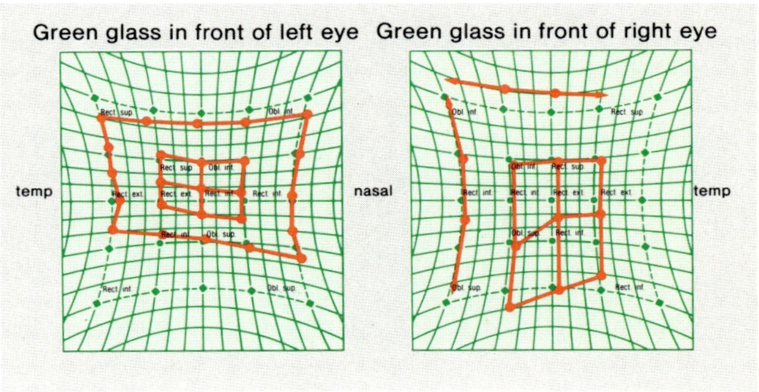

Green glass in front of left eye   Green glass in front of right eye

Fig. 3.11 Hess chart recorded soon after a left blow-out fracture.

Subjective improvement can be monitored by recording the field of binocular single vision; this test is carried out on a perimeter machine that is normally used for measuring visual fields. In this test both eyes are kept open and the patient follows a target from the centre outwards in each meridian until double vision occurs; this point is then marked on the chart.

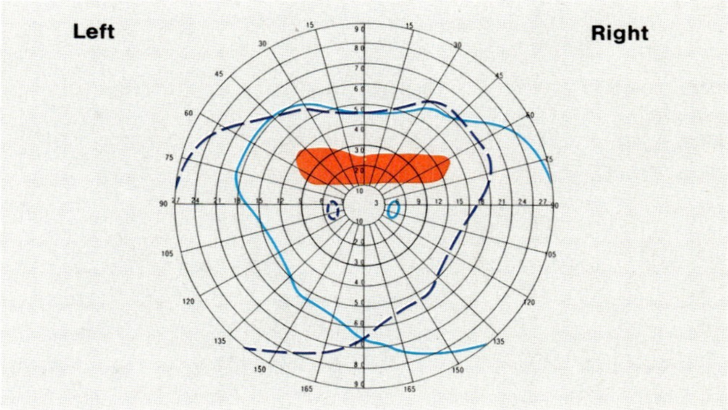

Left   Right

Fig. 3.12 Field of binocular single vision in the same patient.

Conservative versus surgical management

As many patients improve rapidly during the first few days, immediate surgical intervention is not indicated. Over the years, the attitude towards surgical intervention has changed: a policy of conservative management was followed by a period of enthusiastic intervention in all cases; this led to a number of complications and was followed by a period when early intervention was considered inadvisable. The current position advocates early intervention in selected cases: if the indications for surgery are present, this is best carried out between five and ten days after injury.

Indications for surgery in a pure blow-out fracture

1. Double vision in the primary position or on depression persisting 5 days or more.

2. Enophthalmos greater than 2 mm.

3. Obvious retraction of the globe from incarceration.

4. Large 'hanging drop' on x-ray.

The surgical approach is varied. The orbital floor may be exposed from below with a Caldwell-Luc operation, which enters the maxillary sinus via the vestibule of the mouth (see Fig.3.22). The orbital floor is then supported with an antral pack. The disadvantages of this procedure are the risk of chronic maxillary sinusitis, a higher failure rate in correcting diplopia and less reduction of enophthalmos.

Most surgeons have given up this approach in favour of an approach from above, although in some cases, particularly with large defects, a combined approach may be necessary.

The approach from above is by an incision through the junction between the lower lid and the cheek; the periosteum of the infraorbital rim is incised and elevated allowing access to the floor. The orbital tissues are held back with a malleable retractor, allowing a view of tissues herniating into a fracture line.

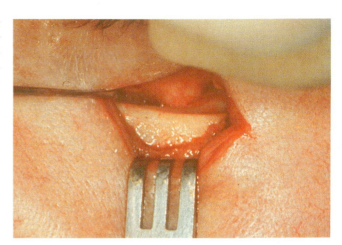

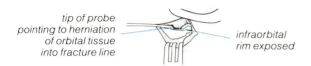

tip of probe pointing to herniation of orbital tissue into fracture line

infraorbital rim exposed

Fig. 3.13 Surgical exposure of the orbital floor from above. By courtesy of Mr. M.J.C. Wake.

Gentle traction is then exerted to bring the herniating tissue back into the orbit. No undue force should be applied, particularly if the inferior rectus muscle itself is incarcerated. Further damage at this stage may convert double vision on upward gaze only to problems with downward gaze as well.

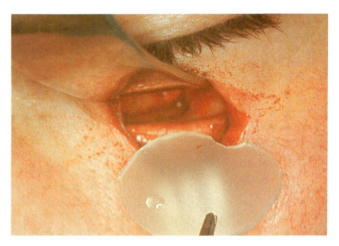

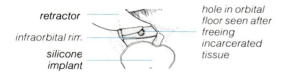

retractor

infraorbital rim.

silicone implant

hole in orbital floor seen after freeing incarcerated tissue

Fig. 3.14 Incarcerated tissue freed from the fracture. By courtesy of Mr. M.J.C. Wake.

This approach also allows repair of the floor with a variety of substances, such as bone wax, fascia lata strips, or silicone plates. The latter should be cut to fit easily into the floor space, then wired anteriorly after drilling holes through the infraorbital rim to prevent extrusion of the implant.

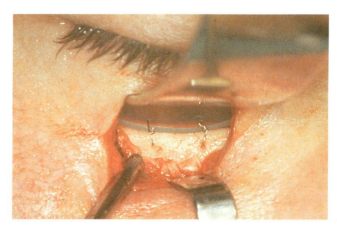

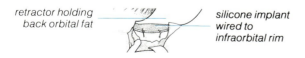

retractor holding back orbital fat

silicone implant wired to infraorbital rim

Fig. 3.15 Silicone plate wired in position. By courtesy of Mr. M.J.C. Wake.

Complications of this procedure include infection or extrusion of the implant, but cases have been recorded with retrobulbar haemorrhage and optic nerve damage; haemostasis should be meticulously performed and pressure dressings should be avoided.

Postoperatively there may be little change in the diplopia, or it may even be worse. A slow improvement occurs over several weeks or months, and is monitored by orthoptic testing as outlined earlier (page 3.5). During the period of recovery, prism lenses may be required to maintain comfortable binocular vision. Ultimately a stable position is reached, and any residual ocular motility problem may need further treatment with strabismus surgery (see page 10.6).

Fractures of the Zygoma

The classical tripartite fracture of the zygoma breaks at three points: the fronto-zygomatic arch is fractured at the suture line; the rim fractures in line with the infra-orbital foramen and the zygomatic arch fractures near the body of the zygoma. The isolated fragment may not be displaced, and in this case no treatment is required. *Backward displacement* can occur, but there is rarely any displacement of the globe or permanent restriction of eye movement.

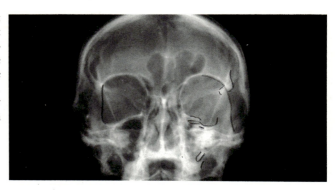

Fig. 3.16 X-ray of a left zygomatic fracture (right and left zygomas highlighted). By courtesy of Mr. M.J.C. Wake.

Downward displacement with rotation may occur by hinging of either the lateral or medial side; lateral hinging displaces the orbital septum downwards with retraction of the lower eyelid, but the position of the globe is not altered. Medial hinging may allow the globe to drop as well if the fronto-zygomatic arch is fractured above the line of attachment of the suspensory ligament of Lockwood. Either type of fracture may be associated with extensive disruption of the orbital floor.

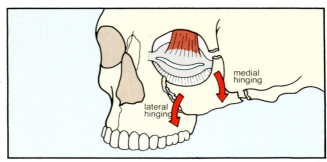

Fig.3.17 Lateral and medial hinging of a zygomatic fracture.

Initially, swelling of the face obscures the injury, but palpation of the infraorbital rim may reveal a step and the affected cheek is flattened. Infraorbital anaesthesia is common. Medial hinging with downward displacement of the lid and globe results in asymmetry of the face, but double vision is usually transient, unless there is an associated blow-out fracture.

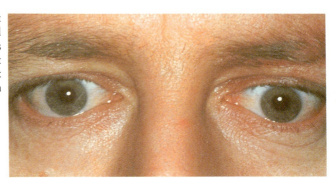

Fig. 3.18 Downward displacement and depression of the left eye in a combined zygomatic and blow-out fracture. By courtesy of Mr. M.J.C. Wake.

The surgical management is the province of the maxillo-facial surgeon; reduction is delayed for a few days to allow the oedema to subside, and the fragment is elevated by a temporal approach and impacted in its normal position. Entrapment of tissues may require exploration of the fronto-zygomatic fracture line and subsequent wiring. If necessary, the orbital floor can then be explored.

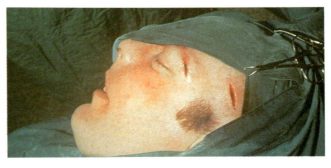

Fig. 3.19 Incisions for reduction and wiring of the above injury. By courtesy of Mr. M.J.C. Wake.

Successful surgery corrects the depression of the globe by restoring the position of Lockwood's ligament and reducing herniation of orbital tissue into the antrum. Some residual defect of ocular motility is common, and secondary strabismus surgery will be required if double vision persists in the primary position or on depression.

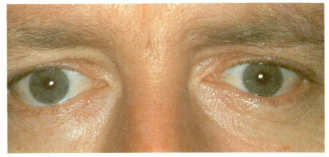

Fig. 3.20 Improved appearance and function after elevating the fractured zygoma and repairing the left orbital floor. By courtesy of Mr. M.J.C. Wake.

If the body of the zygoma is unstable or there are multiple fragments, external splinting may be required. If this is not possible, open reduction with interosseous wiring is performed. There may be an associated blow-out fracture of the orbital floor (see page 3.3), and if the zygoma has been splinted or wired, the floor can be directly explored from above.

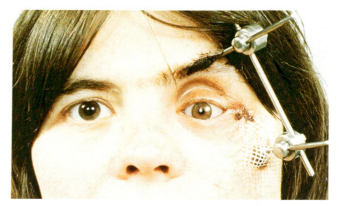

Fig. 3.21 External splinting of a comminuted left zygoma.

Extensive disruption of the orbital floor is common, and the orbital contents need support with a silicone plate (see page 3.6). Where no floor remains, additional support from below is required via a Caldwell-Luc operation. This procedure opens the maxillary antrum from the vestibule of the mouth, allowing access to the disrupted orbital floor.

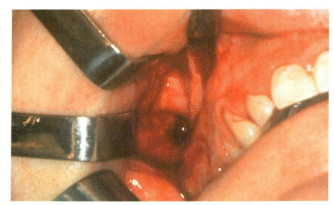

Fig. 3.22 Caldwell-Luc approach to the left orbital floor. By courtesy of Mr. M.J.C. Wake.

An antral pack or polyethylene pillar is introduced to support the silicone plate for a period of three to six weeks. During this period the bony floor reforms from periosteal fragments. Antral packs should not be used if the comminuted zygoma has not been securely fixed, otherwise displacement may occur. Infection is a common problem necessitating removal.

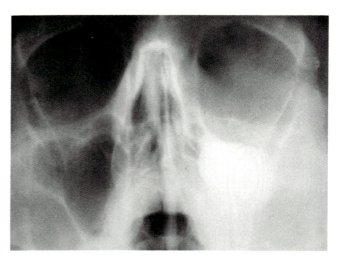

Fig.3.23 X-ray showing a left antral pack supporting an orbital floor fracture. By courtesy of Mr. M.J.C. Wake.

Untreated, this injury leaves a poor cosmetic appearance but double vision is rare unless the displacement is gross or there has been an associated blow-out fracture. After two or three weeks a displaced zygoma is firmly united, and reduction may be extremely difficult at this stage if not impossible.

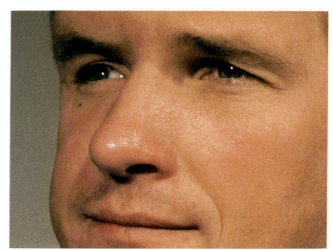

3.8

Fig.3.24 An untreated right zygomatic fracture, showing flattening of the cheek. By courtesy of Mr. M.J.C. Wake.

Recognition of the extent of these injuries is important as airway problems and intracranial complications may be present. A full neurological assessment is essential.

The ophthalmologist will rarely be involved in the early management of these patients, except in those cases where contusion or rupture of the globe has occurred.

Naso-orbital Fractures

A moderate blow to the region of the nose causes collapse of the nasal bones and outward displacement of the frontal processes of the maxillae. The medial canthus is often disinserted along with a fragment of lacrimal bone, resulting in a widening of the inter-palpebral distance and rounding of the inner canthus.

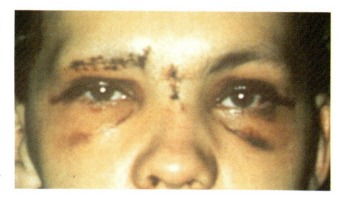

Fig.3.25 Traumatic telecanthus from a naso-orbital fracture. By courtesy of Mr. M.J.C. Wake.

The repair involves transnasal wiring of the displaced canthal ligaments and splinting of the displaced nasal bones. Fractures without any laceration in this region rarely cause disruption of lacrimal drainage, and epiphora is an uncommon complication.

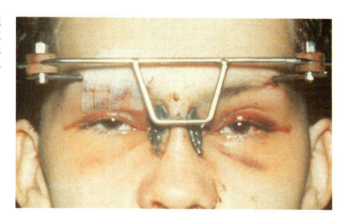

Fig. 3.26 Transnasal wiring and splints for the above injury. By courtesy of Mr. M.J.C. Wake.

A more severe blow to this region results in collapse of the ethmoidal sinuses as well as the nose, and fragments may be driven up to penetrate the anterior cranial fossa resulting in rhinorrhoea. Clear fluid coming from the nose, increased by coughing should arouse suspicion of leaking cerebrospinal fluid; confirmation is obtained by estimating the low protein and high sugar content of the fluid using an appropriate indicator strip. In these more major injuries, immediate surgical reduction may not be possible because of neurological complications; systemic antibiotics are required during this period and the CSF leak often seals spontaneously. Once the general condition is stable, repair can be undertaken. Open reduction with interosseous wiring may be more effective than transnasal wiring in preventing late complications.

Late complications

These concern the ophthalmologist because obstruction of the nasolacrimal duct is common in these more extensive injuries, resulting in a mucocele and recurrent dacryocystitis. Inadequate repair of the medial ligament leaves an unsightly appearance. Surgical treatment is difficult because of the bony deformity and is best carried out by a maxillofacial surgeon. Some improvement can be gained by a dacryocystectomy if reconstruction cannot be performed.

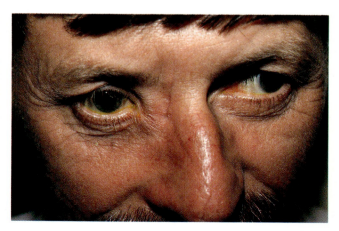

Fig. 3.27 Late appearance of a right naso-orbital fracture.

These depressed fractures always arise from a severe direct blow to the region concerned; the underlying globe is displaced and proptosed, and often suffers severe injury.

In *supraorbital fractures*, the globe is displaced downwards; fragments of bone projecting into the orbit may cause ptosis from damage to the underlying levator muscle and defective elevation from damage to the superior rectus muscle.

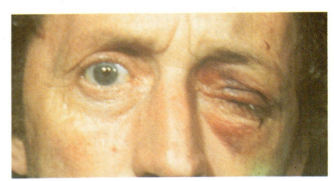

Fig. 3.28 Supraorbital fracture with displacement of the left eye. By courtesy of Mr. M.J.C. Wake.

If the fracture extends to involve the roof of the orbit, the dura can be damaged resulting in a leak of cerebrospinal fluid, or a direct communication may be opened between a sinus and the intracranial cavity. There is a risk of meningitis, and antibiotic cover should be given. A severe head injury prevents early reduction of the fracture until the neurological condition is stable. A craniotomy may be required for damage to the orbital roof, particularly if a dural fistula persists.

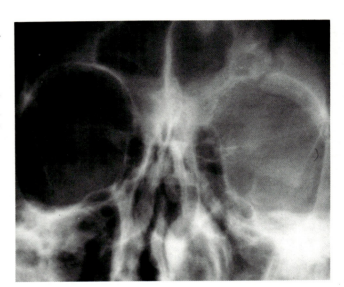

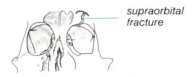

supraorbital fracture

Fig. 3.29 X-ray of the above injury. By courtesy of Mr. M.J.C. Wake.

A blow of sufficient force to fracture the *lateral orbital wall* usually causes severe ocular damage, and is accompanied by orbital haemorrhage causing proptosis. The globe may be ruptured or the optic nerve evulsed.

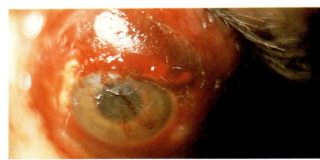

Fig. 3.30 Haemorrhagic proptosis with optic nerve evulsion in a lateral orbital wall fracture.

The management of these severe injuries often involves the close co-operation of many surgical disciplines. The ophthalmologist is required to manage any underlying ocular injury and any residual disturbance of ocular motility.

Raised intraorbital pressure

The orbit is a closed cavity limited anteriorly by the orbital septum; a displaced fracture may reduce the orbital volume, and tissue oedema and haemorrhage lead to a further rise of intraorbital pressure. This embarrasses the venous circulation, which in turn promotes more oedema, leading to a vicious circle. If the patient complains of progressive visual deterioration and no other ocular injury has been found, the fundus should be examined for signs of embarrassment to the retinal circulation. Congested retinal veins and pulsation or closure of the central retinal artery is an indication for emergency decompression of the orbit. An incision is made below the eyebrow, keeping to the medial side to avoid damaging the lacrimal gland; the incision is spread upwards beneath the supraorbital rim to open the orbital septum, taking care to avoid damaging the underlying levator muscle and the superior oblique pulley (see Fig.3.32). This allows gradual extravasation of oedema fluid and relieves the compression until reduction of the fracture can be carried out.

Lacerations breaching the orbital septum may be accompanied by haemorrhage and damage to the periocular tissues. The commonest occurs superiorly and may damage the orbital septum, the underlying levator muscle or the tendon of the superior oblique. Retention of an orbital foreign body may give rise to a chronic granuloma. The management of these injuries has been discussed in Chapter 2 (page 2.7).

More extensive lacerations of orbital tissues may be accompanied by contusion with orbital haemorrhage and raised intraorbital pressure. Urgent exploration will be required if the ophthalmic circulation is compromised. As an emergency measure acetazolamide 500 mg may be given by a slow intravenous injection, as reduction of intraocular pressure may maintain the patency of the central retinal artery.

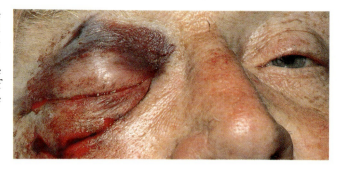

Fig. 3.31 Orbital laceration and proptosis with closure of the right central retinal artery.

The orbital pressure may be reduced by incising the orbital septum at a point away from the area of damage before exploring the wound. Active bleeding from damage to the ethmoidal vessels requires identification and ligation, and the orbital septum should not be closed during repair in case further haemorrhage occurs.

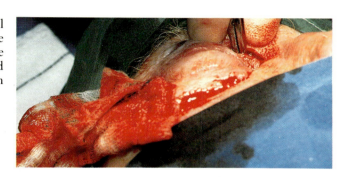

Fig. 3.32 Opening the orbital septum in the above injury.

Optic Nerve Damage

Orbital injuries are usually caused by falling onto a pointed object; a compound orbital fracture may be present. In some patients the external evidence of injury can be minimal. Direct damage to the optic nerve may occur resulting in immediate loss of vision.

If the nerve has been damaged posterior to the entry of the central retinal artery, the initial appearance of the optic disc is normal; optic atrophy develops after three weeks.

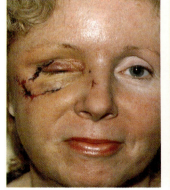 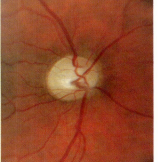

Fig.3.33 left Three weeks after compound fracture and deep laceration of the right orbit.
Fig.3.33 right Optic atrophy affecting the right eye.

If the optic nerve is damaged close to the globe, the retinal circulation will be impaired and the fundus shows signs of gross retinal ischaemia.

In both cases, an afferent pupil defect will be present.

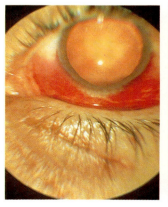 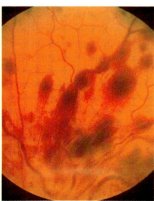

Fig.3.34 left External injury from a finger poked in the eye.
Fig.3.34 right Proximal optic nerve damage with retinal infarction.

CAUTION

Falling onto pointed objects such as pencils or knitting needles is a common injury in children. The history is often unreliable and external evidence of penetration may be minimal. There can be a tiny skin laceration in the eyelids, but if the point has penetrated via the conjunctival fornix, the entry wound may not be obvious. Injury to the optic nerve may occur (see page 3.11), or the roof of the orbit may be penetrated. A careful ophthalmic and neurological examination should be carried out, and x-ray examination is essential to exclude retention of a foreign body or penetration of the orbital roof.

Penetration of the lower eyelid or conjunctival fornix is most likely to be associated with optic nerve damage. A severe reduction in vision occurs, but this may be difficult to assess in infants; optic nerve damage is confirmed by the presence of an afferent pupil defect. Initially the fundus appears normal or there may be mild commotio retinae (see page 5.15), but optic atrophy develops within a few weeks. No treatment is effective and it is important to give a guarded visual prognosis. In a child a divergent squint will rapidly develop.

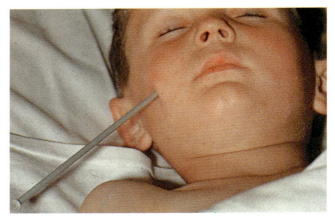

Fig.3.35 Knitting needle penetrating the right orbit and cranium. By courtesy of Mr. J.B. Garston.

Penetration of the upper lid or superior conjunctival fornix may be complicated by penetration of the orbital roof or cavernous sinus. Serious intracranial complications may develop, particularly if foreign material has been retained. Increasing drowsiness and neck stiffness should suggest the development of meningitis or a cerebral abscess, while increasing proptosis and restriction of eye movements accompanied by fever should suggest retention of an intraorbital foreign body or even cavernous sinus thrombosis. Neurosurgical treatment is required without delay.

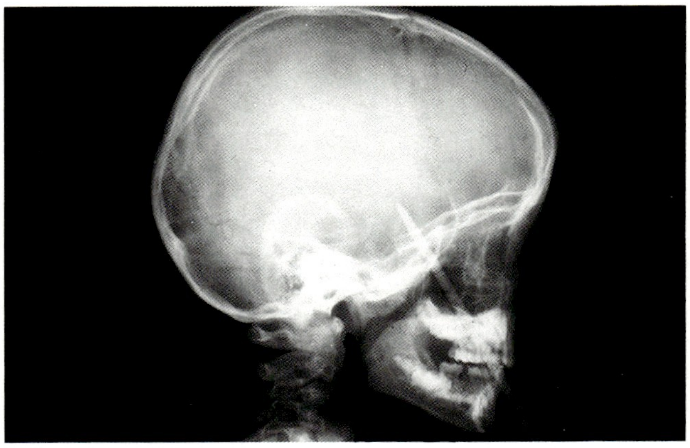

Fig.3.36 X-ray of the above injury showing penetration of the orbital roof. By courtesy of Mr. J.B. Garston.

Orbital Foreign Bodies

The commonest orbital foreign body encountered in ophthalmic practice is a ballistic missile, usually a lead pellet from an air-rifle. Severe ocular contusion is always present (see page 5.15), but occasionally the globe is ruptured (see page 6.28). A double perforation is common, and the pellet is usually lying outside the eye within the orbit or lodged in the paranasal sinuses.

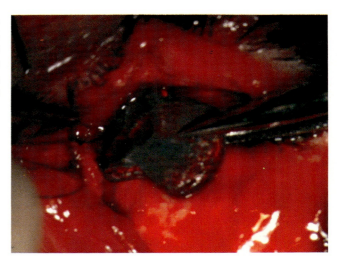

Fig. 3.37 Flattened lead pellet in the orbit, which has caused double perforation of the globe.

The immediate treatment is mainly concerned with the management of the contusion or penetrating injury. If the pellet is visible it can be removed, but if it is located more deeply in the orbit it is best left alone. Removal is unnecessary as the pellet becomes encapsulated, and infection does not occur because of heat sterilisation generated by air-friction.

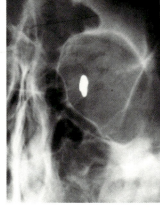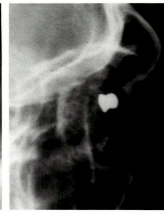

Fig. 3.38 Straight and lateral x-rays of a flattened lead pellet in the orbit that has caused a double perforation of the globe (see Fig. 3.37).

Splinters of wood

Injuries from falling onto bamboo canes or from chips of wood flying up while using an axe may result in retention of a piece of wood within the orbit. It is wise to explore all such injuries under anaesthesia when the history suggests contamination of the wound with organic material.

If the foreign body is not identified and removed soon after injury, an acute orbital cellulitis may develop and produce alarming proptosis with marked systemic toxicity. This may not occur if antibiotic treatment is given prophylactically, but the retained foreign body may then lead to granuloma formation and fluctuating proptosis.

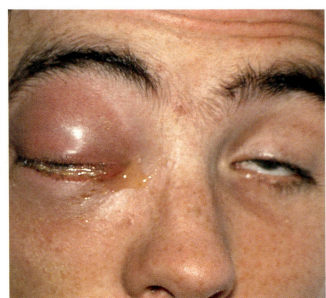

Fig. 3.39 Acute orbital cellulitis complicating a wood chip in the right orbit. By courtesy of Miss E.E. Kritzinger.

Recognition of such an injury may be difficult as the foreign body is often radiolucent, but careful palpation through the eyelid may detect the fragment, or indentation of the globe may be visible on fundus examination. If there is no foreign body visible on x-ray examination, a computerised axial tomogram should be performed. This can confirm the presence of a wood particle and help identify its location.

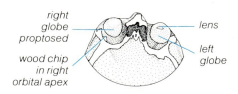

right globe proptosed — lens
wood chip in right orbital apex — left globe

Fig. 3.40 CAT scan showing a wooden foreign body at the orbital apex in the above injury. By courtesy of Miss E.E. Kritzinger.

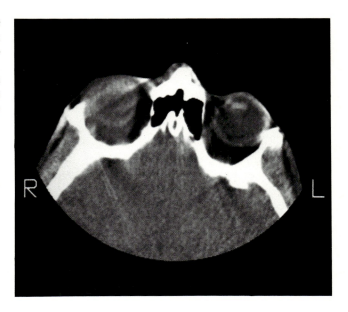

If acute orbital cellulitis is present and is not responding to antibiotic therapy, an emergency orbital decompression is carried out to open the orbital septum. It may not be possible to remove the foreign body at this stage, but decompression allows drainage of pus and better penetration of antibiotic treatment. Once the infection is controlled, an elective exploration of the orbit can be performed to remove the foreign body.

3.13

Orbital Apex Syndrome

Acute proptosis may complicate base of skull fractures involving the superior orbital fissure, or may occur in the absence of a fracture after repeated blows to the orbit. Haemorrhage involving the structures at the apex of the orbit leads to oculomotor palsies; the marked proptosis and mechanical restriction of lid and eye movements masks this in the early stages, but third nerve involvement is indicated by an efferent pupil defect (non-reactive to direct and consensual stimulation).

In the early stages, vision should be monitored to detect any progressive deterioration from raised intra-orbital pressure which may require decompression (see page 3.10); the Visual Evoked Potential is useful in monitoring optic nerve function (see page 3.15). Computerised axial tomography is essential in this injury to exclude an acute subperiosteal haematoma of the roof of the orbit. If present, simple aspiration of blood via the upper lid gives immediate relief.

If no localised haematoma is present and optic nerve function is not threatened, conservative treatment is followed. Strangulation of the conjunctival circulation leads to marked oedema and prolapse over the lid margins (see Fig. 3.41). Corneal sensation may be reduced, and there is a risk of exposure with dryness and secondary infection. The eye must be protected by liberal applications of antibiotic ointment.

As the proptosis and mechanical restriction of eye movement improve, assessment of oculomotor damage becomes possible. Persisting ptosis and restriction of adduction or vertical eye movements indicate a third nerve palsy; this is a common defect in this syndrome.

Chronic Subperiosteal Haematomas of the Orbit

A similar problem may occasionally occur as a late phenomenon after a head injury associated with a skull fracture. A sudden onset of proptosis with downward or axial displacement of the globe occurs after a definite time interval following the head trauma. The proptosis may increase to give a severe exposure problem, and vision may be threatened by embarrassment to the ophthalmic circulation as described above.

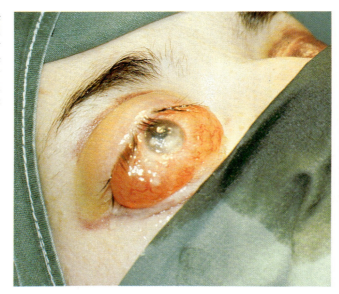

Fig. 3.41 Gross proptosis from a chronic subperiosteal haematoma. By courtesy of Mr. V.H. Smith.

In children the history of a head injury may be uncertain, and the clinical picture can resemble a pseudotumour of the orbit, with recurrent episodes of proptosis. X-ray examination may confirm a fracture involving the base of skull, and bony destruction sometimes involves the orbital roof. Computerised axial tomography will outline the subperiosteal haematoma.

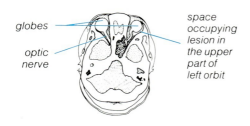

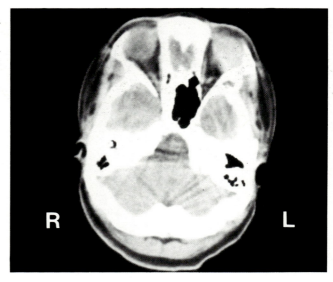

Fig. 3.42 CAT scan of a left subperiosteal haematoma.

In chronic cases or where the diagnosis is uncertain, a lateral orbitotomy may be required; the subdural haematoma may be fluid, but if long-standing, granuloma formation involving the adjacent bone may occur. Evacuation of the clot or granuloma with drainage usually prevents recurrence.

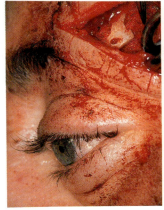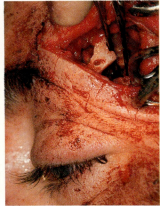

Fig.3.43 left Exploration of a chronic subperiosteal haematoma of the left orbit: the evacuated cavity has been packed to demonstrate the proptosis.
Fig.3.43 right Reduction in the proptosis after complete evacuation. By courtesy of Mr. V.H. Smith.

Intracranial Damage to the Visual Pathways

Severe frontal impacts can cause damage to the canalicular part of the optic nerve; a fracture of the base of the skull or optic canal is present in some cases. Immediate visual loss is the result of shearing forces which damages the microvasculature of the optic nerve; this is irreversible and surgical intervention is not indicated. The optic disc appears normal initially, but visual loss and an afferent pupil defect should suggest the diagnosis. Optic atrophy develops after three weeks.

If vision is present initially, but deteriorates, optic nerve compression may be present from displaced bony fragments or vascular damage may lead to haematoma formation. Spontaneous improvement occurs in a third of patients; transethmoidal decompression of the optic canal has the same success rate and is indicated if tomograms demonstrate clear compression of the optic nerve.

Chiasmal damage also occurs after closed head injuries, but is less common than optic nerve involvement. Higher visual pathway damage accompanies extensive intracranial injuries, but this can only be assessed when there has been some recovery. When concentration permits, improvement can be monitored by serial visual field testing.

Measurement of the Visual Evoked Potential may help confirm optic nerve or visual pathway damage. Simultaneous monitoring of the electro-encephalogram is needed in patients who have had a significant head injury.

The Visual Evoked Potential is a modification of the electro-encephalogram; the response to repeated flash or pattern stimuli is averaged to eliminate background activity. This gives a complex wave form, of which the P2 component is the most consistent; both amplitude and latency are important parameters. The flash response gives an overall indication of visual function, while the pattern response is more sensitive to macula and optic nerve pathology. Higher visual pathway damage can also be detected.

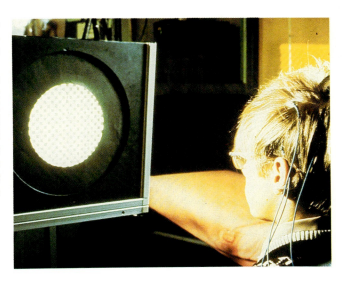

Fig.3.44 Measuring the Visual Evoked Potential. By courtesy of Professor G. Harding.

Ocular Motility Problems

Major head injuries are often associated with damage to the third, fourth and sixth cranial nerves (vide infra). Isolated pupil dilatation with a deteriorating level of consciousness is a serious sign, indicating raised intracranial pressure requiring urgent neurosurgical attention.

Brainstem damage leading to bizarre eye movements with skew deviation, gaze palsies and internuclear ophthalmoplegia are all common after a major head injury with loss of consciousness, while an acute supranuclear palsy will accompany severe frontal lobe damage (the eyes being deviated to the affected side). These signs usually improve as consciousness returns. Cerebellar damage leads to nystagmus and ocular dysmetria, while involvement of the oculomotor pathways results in disorders of saccadic and pursuit movements. In the less severe injuries, weakening of the binocular fusion range and decompensation of a pre-existing muscle imbalance is common.

Persisting problems of ocular motility often interfere with rehabilitation after a major head injury, and orthoptic treatment may be required.

Involvement of these cranial nerves is common after head injuries with or without a fractured skull; they are most commonly associated with a frontal impact. Third nerve involvement is usually unilateral, while fourth and sixth nerve palsies are often bilateral. Recovery occurs over several months and is usually good, but third nerve palsies associated with the orbital apex syndrome (see page 3.14) have a bad prognosis.

Third nerve paresis results in defective adduction, elevation and depression of the affected eye. A divergent squint may be present, which is greater when fixing with the paretic eye. Initially complete ptosis is present and the pupil is dilated from involvement of the parasympathetic innervation; some reaction to direct and consensual light stimulation is usually retained.

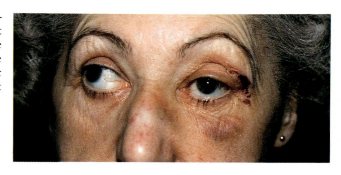

Fig. 3.45 Traumatic left third nerve palsy.

When the third nerve is paralysed, the integrity of the fourth cranial nerve is tested by asking the patient to look down and in; wheel rotation of the globe confirms the function of the superior oblique muscle. Isolated *fourth nerve damage* causes a superior oblique palsy with weakness of depression in adduction (see Fig. 2.26); torsional diplopia occurs, which the patient learns to avoid by tilting the head to the opposite side.

A *sixth nerve palsy* affects the lateral rectus muscle with limitation of abduction resulting in a convergent squint; the patient develops a head turn to the affected side to avoid double vision.

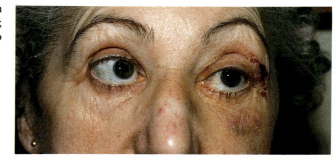

Fig. 3.46 Left sixth nerve palsy accompanying the above injury.

In total third nerve palsies, complete ptosis prevents troublesome diplopia initially, but when this recovers double vision becomes a problem which often persists. Surgical treatment is difficult because several muscles are affected; suppression of the false image usually develops, but continued occlusion for diplopia may be required.

Traumatic third nerve palsies have a high incidence of misdirection of the nerve fibres during recovery; anomalies of eyelid and pupil function are common, with elevation of the eyelid on attempted downgaze and variations in pupil size with eye movement.

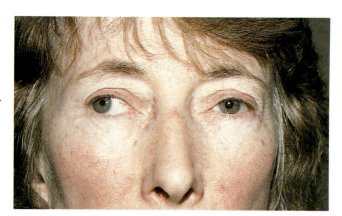

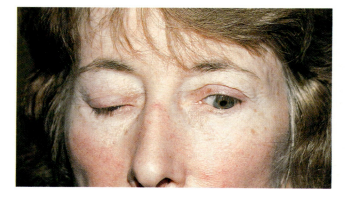

Fig.3.47 upper Incomplete recovery of a left third nerve palsy, with ptosis and pupil enlargement.
Fig.3.47 lower Inappropriate elevation of the left upper lid and pupil constriction on downgaze.

Incomplete recovery of traumatic fourth nerve palsies gives rise to troublesome torsional diplopia on down-gaze, and early surgical treatment is required. Antero-lateral advancement of the anterior portion of the superior oblique tendon is the treatment of choice.

In sixth nerve palsies, a head turn to the affected side helps reduce double vision. Recovery is monitored by orthoptic assessment and repeated Lees screen; binocular vision may be restored with the aid of Fresnel prisms, which can be attached to glasses and reduced in strength as improvement occurs. Late surgical treatment can be considered for persisting defects (see Chapter 10).

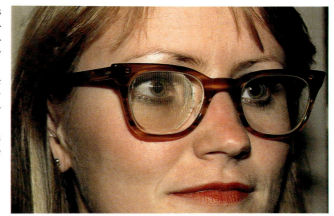

Fig. 3.48 Fresnel prism assisting binocular vision.

Carotico-cavernous Fistula

This complication of a head injury is usually associated with a fractured base of skull; although damage occurs to the intracavernous part of the internal carotid artery at the time of injury, symptoms are not immediate and may develop several days or weeks later. The less common ruptures from stab wounds through the orbit usually give rise to immediate proptosis.

The patient complains of severe headache and sudden onset of noises in the head when the internal carotid artery ruptures into the cavernous sinus. The eye on the affected side becomes progressively proptosed with restriction of eye movements, and pulsating exophthalmos is often present; involvement of the other eye occurs in a percentage of patients from intercommunication of the cavernous sinuses. A cranial bruit synchronous with the pulsating exophthalmos may be audible.

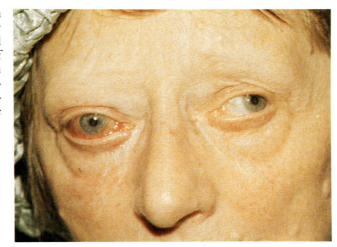

Fig.3.49 Proptosis from a right carotico-cavernous fistula.

Progressive visual deterioration and ocular pain may develop. Bright red engorgement of the episcleral vessels occurs as arterialised blood fills the venous system; a fall in perfusion pressure of the ophthalmic artery and increased venous pressure leads to ocular ischaemia, with a hypoxic retinopathy, uveitis and anterior segment ischaemia.

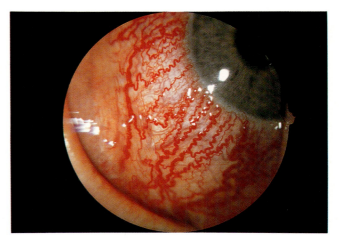

Fig. 3.50 Arterial engorgement of episcleral vessels from a carotico-cavernous fistula.

The visual outcome is poor both with conservative treatment and with surgical attempts to close the fistula; treatment of uveitis, glaucoma and secondary complications of retinal ischaemia may help, and ultimately the vision may stabilise or recover by spontaneous thrombosis of the fistula. Eyes threatened by severe ischaemia and anterior segment necrosis are unlikely to benefit from a surgical attempt at closure, and these procedures have a high morbidity and mortality risk.

Facial Nerve Damage

The facial nerve may be damaged in a head injury and unless rapid improvement occurs there may be a risk of corneal exposure. If the patient is unconscious the eyelids should be taped shut to prevent exposure, or a temporary central tarsorrhaphy can be performed with 1 metric (5/0) nylon. If no recovery occurs and corneal sensation is also impaired, a permanent lateral tarsorrhaphy will be required. If corneal sensation is intact and a good Bell's phenomenon is present, conservative treatment with ocular lubricants and a side-shield on spectacles can be tried; persistent corneal staining is an indication for lateral tarsorrhaphy.

Persisting paralysis of the orbicularis will lead to ectropion of the lower lid and contracture of the upper lid; if there is no sign of any recovery within three months, facial nerve transplants or craniofacial anastomoses may be considered. If conservative treatment is adopted, and recovery is incomplete by twelve months, surgical reconstruction should be carried out. The lower lid can be supported with a silastic thread or fascial sling attached to the medial and lateral palpebral ligaments, and the upper lid is stretched by a small gold implant sutured to the tarsal plate or a Morel-Fatio spring to prevent the subsequent contracture of the unapposed levator muscle. Mild degrees of ectropion affecting the lower lid can be managed by a lid shortening procedure and a small medial tarsorrhaphy together with excision of an ellipse of conjunctiva adjacent to the punctum. This helps to prevent chronic watering of the eye by reapposing the lower lid and punctum.

Details of these techniques are beyond the scope of this book, and reference should be made to standard texts on Plastic Surgery.

Indirect Ocular Damage from Head Injuries

The abrupt deceleration forces that occur during a head injury cause a dynamic disturbance of the vitreous within the eye; this may precipitate a posterior vitreous detachment and a retinal tear in patients with pre-existing lattice degeneration of the retina. This is more common in myopic individuals, and is accompanied by light flashes and floaters for a few days; progressive field loss and visual failure indicates the development of a retinal detachment. Early surgical treatment is required as central vision may not recover once affected, and the success rate is greater in the early stages.

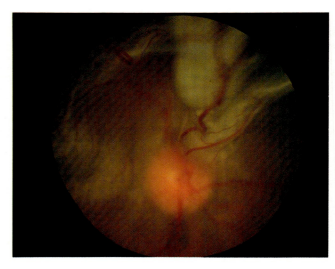

Fig.3.51 Retinal detachment after a head injury.

Vitreous haemorrhage may accompany a traumatic sub-arachnoid haemorrhage, or occur in non-accidental injury in childhood (vide infra); if dense, this will leave a permanent opacity in the vitreous gel. In bilateral cases, early vitrectomy will need to be considered.

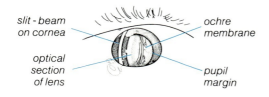

slit - beam
on cornea

ochre
membrane

optical
section
of lens

pupil
margin

Fig. 3.52 Dense vitreous haemorrhage following head trauma.

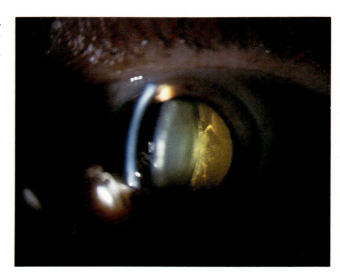

Careful ocular examination is required, as direct injury is a more likely cause of vitreous haemorrhage. A Visual Evoked Potential (see page 3.15) will help confirm the integrity of the visual pathways, while an electroretinogram and ultrasonography (page 7.4) will detect the presence of retinal detachment.

Non-accidental Injury in Children

Non-accidental injury in children from repeated head shaking or concussion is an important cause of vitreous haemorrhage, retinal and optic nerve damage. The children are usually under the age of two years, with evidence of neglect and multiple soft tissue injuries; x-ray examination reveals fractures at different stages of repair. If non-accidental injury is suspected, the child should be kept in hospital while investigations are carried out and appropriate action is taken.

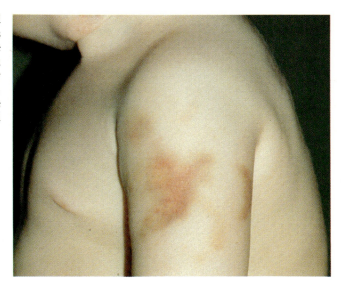

Fig. 3.53 Multiple bruising and neglect in a battered baby. By courtesy of Dr. Stephen Rose.

Ophthalmic signs include periorbital bruising, signs of previous haemorrhage such as organised vitreous or macular scars, fresh preretinal or subretinal haemorrhages, and evidence of optic nerve or visual pathway damage. Cortical blindness is not uncommon, which can be confirmed by the absence of the Visual Evoked Potential.

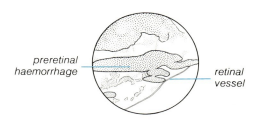

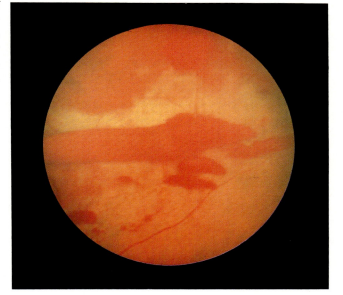

Fig. 3.54 Preretinal haemorrhages as seen in non-accidental injury. By courtesy of Mr. S.S.F. Munro.

The visual consequences for these children are serious. Optic atrophy and retinal scarring involving the macular region are common, resulting in poor vision and nystagmus; partial-sight education is usually required. Cortical blindness is more serious and is associated with cerebral palsy and epilepsy. Education for blindness may be required.

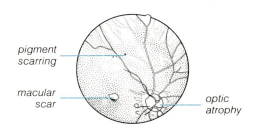

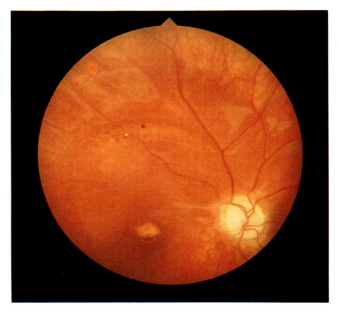

Fig. 3.55 Optic atrophy and retinal scarring following battering in infancy.

Retinal changes may be associated with general injuries and will affect vision if the macula is involved. Attempted strangulation and compression injuries of the chest give rise to multiple preretinal haemorrhages and cotton wool spots close to the optic disc, while fat embolism from fracture of a long bone causes scattered micro-infarcts of the retina, with cotton wool spots sometimes surrounded by a halo of haemorrhage. The ocular changes develop a few days after injury and usually resolve, but early pulmonary or cerebral involvement carries a high mortality.

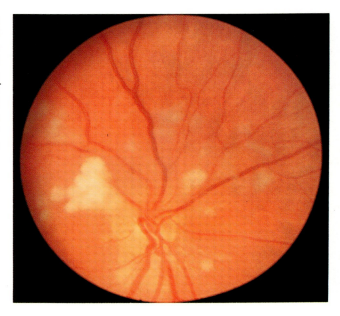

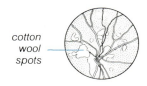

Fig. 3.56 Fat embolism of the retina.

Patients who survive electrocution have transient blindness which generally recovers within hours or minutes after the injury; macular oedema with central scotomata may be present, and some patients develop permanent retinal changes and optic atrophy. Bilateral cataract formation is common, developing weeks or months after injury.

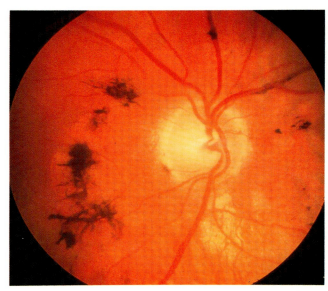

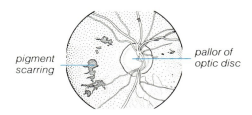

Fig. 3.57 Progressive retinal pigmentation after electrocution. By courtesy of Mr. S.S.F. Munro.

Central visual loss is seen after a solar burn from observing an eclipse with inadequate protection; a retinal burn develops at the macula, resulting in a small positive scotoma and distortion of vision. A small punched-out scar affecting the macula remains, and vision is permanently affected.

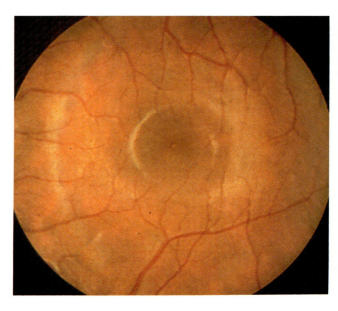

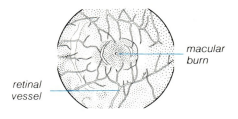

Fig. 3.58 Eclipse burn of the macula. By courtesy of Mr. S.S.F. Munro.

4

Burns to the Eye and Periocular Tissues

BURNS TO THE EYE AND PERIOCULAR TISSUES

The extent and severity of the injury will vary with the cause, but certain common patterns are observed. Superficial injuries from radiation and minor chemical irritants are discussed in Chapter 1 (pages 1.20–22), while this chapter will consider in detail the presentation and management of chemical and thermal burns.

Immediate Treatment

Chemical burns

The urgency of the immediate treatment for chemical burns needs further emphasis: progressive damage may occur from the continued presence of a chemical agent, particularly if it is alkaline. Its nature should be identified from the history and emergency irrigation repeated, continuing for as long as there is any possibility of chemical action. For caustic burns continuous irrigation with compound sodium lactate solution (Hartmann's solution) is carried out, using a drip-set and a speculum or irrigating contact lens; 5 ml of 0.1% bromothymol blue can be added to 500 ml of the irrigating solution to act as an indicator. A neutral solution is green; strong alkalis turn the effluent blue, while acids make the colour more yellow. This indicator system is most useful in fresh lime or mortar burns.

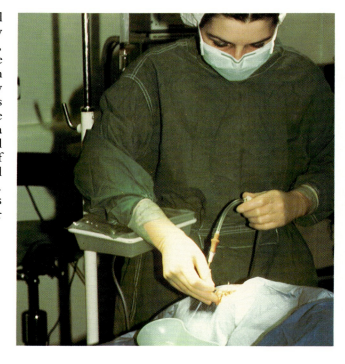

Fig.4.1 Irrigation system using bromothymol blue.

After irrigating lime burns, any solid particles or debris should be removed with a moist cotton wool bud or non-toothed forceps. Irrigation of fresh lime burns with sodium edetate solution 0.4% should be avoided, as this converts calcium hydroxide to sodium hydroxide giving a rise of pH. This solution may be used for patients presenting 24 hours after injury, when the lime has been converted to calcium carbonate.

Thermal burns

With thermal burns the damage is done at the time of injury; molten metal burns form a cast which needs to be gently removed with sterile blunt forceps after instilling local anaesthetic drops.

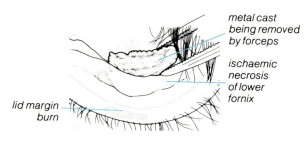

metal cast being removed by forceps

ischaemic necrosis of lower fornix

lid margin burn

Fig.4.2 Removal of a molten metal cast.

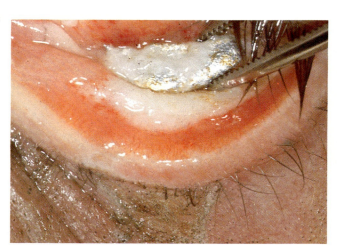

In any severe burn, blepharospasm and marked lid oedema may make immediate treatment and subsequent assessment difficult, and general anaesthesia may be required.

After completing the emergency treatment, the extent of damage to the eye and to the surrounding tissues is assessed and future management planned.

The Pattern of Injury in Ocular Burns

Chemical burns

The severity of a chemical burn will depend on its nature, concentration and duration of contact with the tissues. Gases are less noxious than liquids or solid particles. The nature of the chemical determines the penetration of tissues and their reaction.

Acid burns

In general, acids coagulate the surface creating a barrier against further penetration, and the damage is mainly confined to the surface tissues.

Car battery explosions are the commonest cause of acid burns; although the chemical injury is usually superficial, it is often bilateral, and the explosive nature of the injury may result in contusion or perforation of the globe.

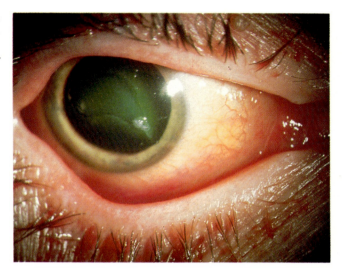

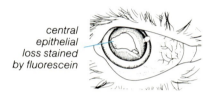

central epithelial loss stained by fluorescein

Fig.4.3 Superficial chemical burn from a car battery explosion.

Injury from concentrated acids is less common, but occurs in industrial accidents or from assault. Concentrated sulphuric acid is particularly harmful because of its dehydrating action.

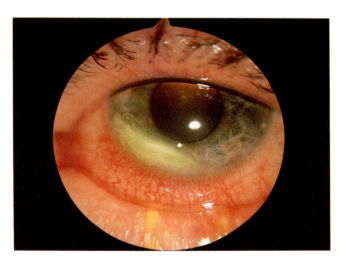

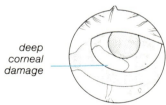

deep corneal damage

Fig.4.4 Localised corneal necrosis from concentrated sulphuric acid.

Alkali burns

Many alkalis and hydrofluoric acid are lipid soluble and rapidly penetrate the tissues; their effect is both widespread and deep. They have a prolonged effect by being held in the tissues, causing continuing damage *(progressive burns)*.

Lime or mortar are common causes of an alkali burn, and are particularly harmful as particles may be trapped in the fornices causing continuing action.

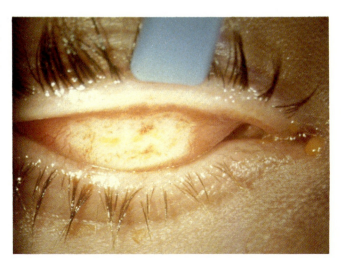

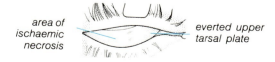

area of ischaemic necrosis

everted upper tarsal plate

Fig.4.5 Lime burn showing damage to the upper tarsal plate.

The stronger alkalis such as caustic soda or liquid ammonia penetrate very rapidly and cause severe injury. Deep penetration with extensive limbal involvement leads to anterior segment ischaemia. In these injuries prolonged irrigation is important.

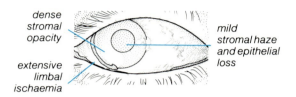

dense stromal opacity

mild stromal haze and epithelial loss

extensive limbal ischaemia

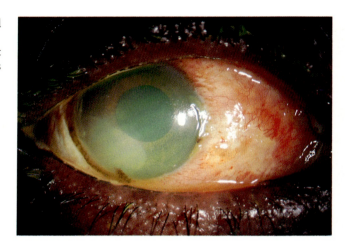

Fig.4.6 Caustic soda burn with deep stromal damage. (See Figs.4.19 and 4.20 for later appearances.)

Molten metal burns

A splash of molten metal is a common industrial injury. The liquid metal will be at a very high temperature, and the extent of damage will depend on the volume that hits the eye. The molten metal remains liquid for long enough to flow into the lower fornix where it forms a cast. Severe necrosis is always present around the site of solidification (see Fig.4.2).

If the splash of molten metal is small, the damage may be quite localised and reflex elevation of the eyes may protect the cornea from injury. If the cornea is involved it is usually the lower half that is affected. Pitting or facetting of the burnt surface indicates a deep, probably full-thickness burn. The line of demarcation between necrotic and viable tissue is clearly shown by the limit of vascular engorgement.

The molten metal will burn the adjacent palpebral surface and eyelid structures, and may spill over the lid margin; these injuries are often associated with *severe eyelid damage*. Occasionally the volume of molten metal is sufficient to fill the conjunctival sac and to cover the skin surface of both lids; full-thickness lid necrosis is likely in addition to a severe ocular burn.

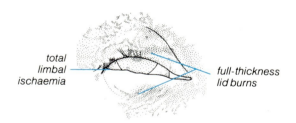

total limbal ischaemia

full-thickness lid burns

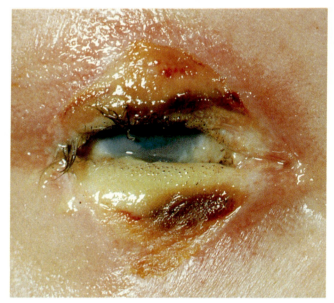

Fig.4.7 Molten metal destruction of eye and lids eight days after burn. By courtesy of Mr. J.P. Gowar.

Assessment of Ocular Burns

Although the pattern of injury varies according to the cause, the nature of the damage is similar for both chemical and thermal burns, and the examination procedure is the same. The initial assessment should start by recording the visual acuity, and should determine the degree of damage to all structures involved.

Pain and lid swelling may make examination difficult, and instillation of benoxinate drops to give local anaesthesia is usually necessary; these drops are painful on instillation, and appreciation of this should be recorded. In severe burns the corneal nerves are destroyed, and the absence of pain with corneal anaesthesia is a bad prognostic sign.

When marked lid swelling is present, particularly with burns involving the skin surface, *sterile lid retractors* should be used to examine the globe. If adequate assessment is not possible after instilling local anaesthetic drops, the examination should be performed under general anaesthesia. In this situation consent should be obtained for full surgical debridement, as described later in this section (see page 4.8).

Damage to the cornea may be superficial, with epithelial oedema or loss; involvement of the underlying stroma results in a varying degree of opacification ranging from mild opalescence to complete loss of transparency. Epithelial loss is demonstrated by vital staining with a drop of 1% fluorescein; surrounding epithelial damage will be demonstrated by 1% rose bengal.

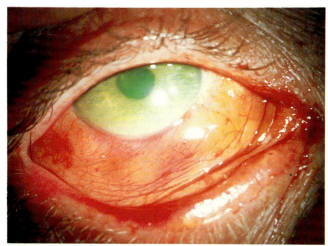

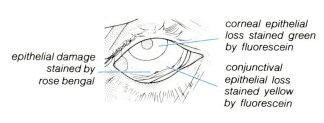

Fig.4.8 Lime burn stained for epithelial damage or loss.

The transparency of the cornea should be recorded; this may be normal, but if it is impaired the ability to distinguish iris details should be noted. The area involved should be carefully charted, including any surface irregularities and the degree of swelling. In deep burns slit-lamp examination will reveal marked stromal swelling with folds in Descemet's membrane.

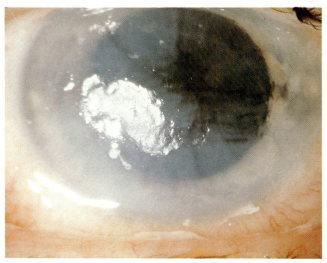

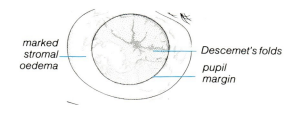

Fig.4.9 Severe corneal burn with stromal oedema.

Damage to the conjunctiva and episcleral tissue may be superficial with hyperaemia, epithelial loss and oedema, leading to pronounced ballooning of the conjunctiva (chemosis). Vital staining will reveal the extent of epithelial damage. In examining the conjunctiva all surfaces should be studied, including both fornices and the inner and outer canthal regions with the eye abducted or adducted respectively. This is particularly important in lime or molten metal burns where fornix damage is common, but may be missed (see Fig.4.5). Particles may also be trapped under the plica semilunaris, causing a localised burn as illustrated.

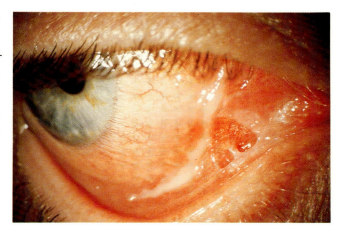

Fig.4.10 Gramoxone burn of the inner canthal region.

More severe injuries lead to *ischaemia of the underlying sclera*, with avascularity and necrosis. The limbus is an important area to look for signs of ischaemia (see Fig.4.12), as this will correlate with deeper damage to the internal structures; the extent of this should be recorded. Deep involvement of both cornea and sclera will be accompanied by signs of *anterior segment ischaemia*; there will be a marked flare and cells in the anterior chamber, and the intraocular pressure will be unstable, initially tending to hypotony, but later swinging to intractable glaucoma.

In severe burns it may not be possible to see through the oedematous cornea, and this always indicates a catastrophic injury; in these patients hyphaema or hypopyon develop after a few days, and a rapidly maturing cataract may occur. Corneal ulceration and perforation is likely to develop in the second week after injury.

After completing the examination, the severity of the burn is classified so that management can be planned and the prognosis evaluated.

Assessing the grade of injury is important in determining subsequent management, particularly in the progressive alkali burns where more radical treatment may be required. The following grading scheme describes the appearance and likely outcome of widespread ocular burns; a better prognosis is expected if the burn is localised.

Grading of ocular damage

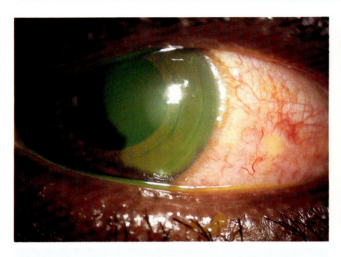

Grade I

Cornea	Epithelial loss only.
Conjunctiva	No ischaemia.
Prognosis	Good: full recovery.

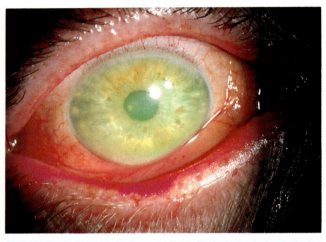

Grade II

Cornea	Some stromal haze but iris visible.
Conjunctiva	Ischaemia less than one third of limbus.
Prognosis	Good : some scarring.

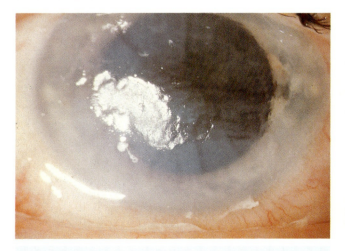

Grade III

Cornea	Widespread stromal haze; iris details obscured.
Conjunctiva	Ischaemia affects one third to half of limbus.
Prognosis	Uncertain: vision impaired; perforation rare.

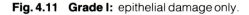

Grade IV

Cornea	Opaque: no view of iris or pupil.
Conjunctiva	Ischaemia greater than half of the limbus.
Prognosis	Poor: expect perforation.

Fig. 4.11 Grade I: epithelial damage only.

Grade III: extensive limbal ischaemia.

Grade II: mild stromal damage and limbal ischaemia.

Grade IV: dense stromal haze with total limbal ischaemia.

Treatment of Ocular Involvement

The aims of treatment are to promote epithelialisation as soon as possible, and to protect the cornea against further damage by exposure or infection during the healing period. Daily conjunctival cultures should be taken to detect the presence of pathogenic organisms, and patients should be nursed in a surgically clean area. General measures include adequate analgesia and sedation as initially the condition may be very painful.

Management of Grade I and II Burns

Most of these injuries will be non-progressive, from acid or thermal burns, but some caustic burns may come in this category.

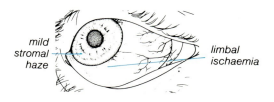

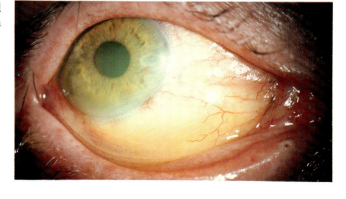

Fig.4.12 Lime burn involving the cornea and inferior fornix.

In this situation it may be helpful to give a subconjunctival injection of the patient's own blood; this helps to separate tissues and acts as a buffer for the noxious agent. The blood is taken in a heparinised syringe, and injected under healthy conjunctiva.

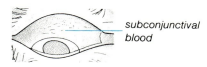

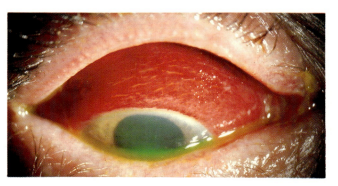

Fig.4.13 Heparinised blood injected via the upper fornix.

Treatment consists of antibiotic drops (10% chloramphenicol in the first instance, changing to an appropriate antibiotic if bacterial colonisation occurs), together with 1% atropine drops b.d. to relieve the pain. Freshly prepared 10% ascorbate drops are prescribed two-hourly (see page 4.9). Initially the eye is covered with a firm pad; once the epithelium has almost healed, dark glasses may be more comfortable.

Grade I injuries will heal quickly, but deeper burns may take one or two weeks to epithelialise.

Fig.4.14 Lime burn one day after injury, showing a large epithelial defect.

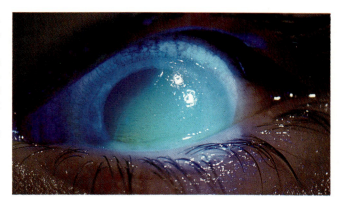

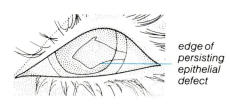

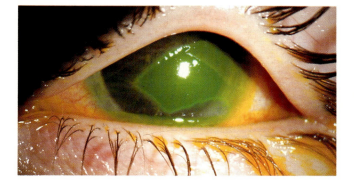

Fig.4.15 Same injury eight days later.

An indolent epithelial defect or recurrent erosions may be a problem. The early use of 10% ascorbate drops two-hourly helps prevent this, but if epithelialisation stops or regresses, 0.5% disodium edetate drops two-hourly are added to the regimen (see page 4.9). A persisting epithelial defect can also be helped by artificial tear drops or a soft contact lens to act as a bandage.

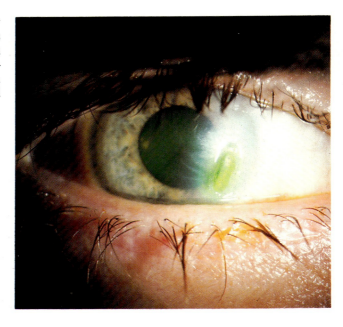

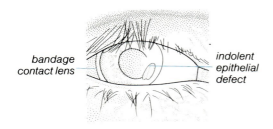

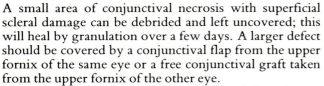

bandage contact lens

indolent epithelial defect

Fig.4.16 Persisting epithelial defect after a lime burn.

A small area of conjunctival necrosis with superficial scleral damage can be debrided and left uncovered; this will heal by granulation over a few days. A larger defect should be covered by a conjunctival flap from the upper fornix of the same eye or a free conjunctival graft taken from the upper fornix of the other eye.

Where there is a full-thickness burn of the sclera or cornea, there may be areas of deep ischaemia sharply demarcated from healthy tissues; this particularly occurs in molten metal burns, and these areas of necrosis will delay healing and promote fibroplasia. Early corneal grafting may be effective both for corneal and scleral damage, using a deep lamellar or penetrating corneal transplant according to the depth of the burn. This reduces subsequent fibroplasia and helps prevent astigmatism, symblepharon or staphyloma formation.

Topical steroids may be helpful in these less severe injuries but should be used with caution: they can be very useful in reducing vascularisation of a damaged cornea, and in ameliorating internal inflammation, but their use may lead to rapid softening of the cornea in the presence of limbal ischaemia.

Management of Grade III and IV Burns

The majority of these burns will be progressive alkali burns, although some molten metal or concentrated acid burns may fall into this category. A conservative approach is usually adopted for the non-progressive burns, but more radical treatment is required for the progressive alkali burns because of retention of the noxious agent in the tissues.

Emergency treatment: Progressive burns

Where conditions permit, a subconjunctival injection of heparinised blood may be a useful emergency measure, and irrigation should be continued for a prolonged period. Many severe alkali burns will require examination and debridement under general anaesthesia, and consent should be obtained for a full surgical procedure.

In these caustic burns, rapid penetration of the alkali into the anterior chamber occurs within seconds, raising the pH of the aqueous. Experimental studies have shown that this rise persists for about two hours. Although some benefit has been demonstrated experimentally by anterior chamber lavage, clinical experience has been disappointing. A simple paracentesis may be of some benefit, and repeated anterior chamber lavage can be performed with a balanced salt solution.

Because these measures have not proved to be very effective, radical surgical treatment has been advocated for all Grade III and IV progressive alkali burns; the aim is to excise the damaged tissues to prevent continued action of the noxious agent, and to remove completely devitalised tissues. To be effective this needs to be carried out within 24 hours of injury, and a very extensive graft may be required; it is important to preserve the donor corneal epithelium, and remove necrotic episcleral tissues close to the limbus. The conjunctiva should be recessed to the insertions of the rectus muscles. After emergency corneal grafting, a similar regimen to that described below is followed.

Further management

As with the less severe burns, treatment is directed to preventing infection; topical antibiotics, mydriatics and ascorbate drops are prescribed (see page 4.7), and the eye is padded. In these severe burns *topical steroids should be avoided*, as rapid melting may occur in the presence of limbal ischaemia.

The initial course of these injuries is deceptive; slow corneal epithelialisation commences, and the appearance may remain unchanged for a few days. Between the fifth and seventh day after injury a sudden worsening occurs, with cessation or sometimes regression of epithelialisation, accompanied by stromal infiltrate and ulceration leading to eventual perforation. In Grade IV burns, hyphaema or hypopyon often develop in the second week after injury, indicating anterior segment destruction and necrosis of tissues. This is often a precursor to retrocorneal membrane formation.

Much experimental work has been carried out to investigate the factors responsible for this. In these full-thickness burns, total cell death of all the involved tissues occurs; subsequent invasion by polymorphonucleocytes commences, leading to direct release of destructive enzymes and plasminogen activator. Experimental work has indicated that immunosuppression with cyclophosphamide reduces the incidence of corneal ulceration by inflammatory cell depletion; this treatment should be considered at the outset in severe bilateral injuries.

Interactions also take place with epithelial cells and invading fibroblasts to release collagenase. Soft contact lenses may be used to promote early epithelialisation, although symblepharon formation may make this impracticable. Both experimental and clinical studies have supported the use of collagenase inhibitors, which should be introduced to the treatment regimen if epithelialisation stops or regresses. Cysteine drops have been recommended, but the preparation is unstable, and it is preferable to use disodium edetate 0.5% drops every two hours until the surface is epithelialised.

Recent experimental work suggests that other mechanisms apart from collagenase may contribute to the breakdown of collagen; direct toxicity from oxygen penetrating the damaged cornea may lead to harmful superoxide radicals accumulating because of the absence of the protective enzyme system, and these may result directly in the depolymerisation of collagen.

In these severely burnt eyes the level of ascorbic acid is reduced; this acts as a scavenger for superoxide radicals, and some protection against ulceration is obtained by using 10% ascorbate drops every 2 hours. This regimen is commenced immediately after injury. Parenteral therapy with Vitamin C is less effective, possibly because of impaired ciliary body function.

Raised intraocular pressure should be controlled by topical and systemic treatment. Pilocarpine is irritating to an inflamed eye, while adrenaline drops cause vaso-constriction and may increase the ischaemia; 0.5% timolol drops b.d. are the treatment of choice locally, while acetazolamide tablets (250 mg) may be used systemically up to four times a day with potassium supplements.

Management of Fornix and Lid Margin Burns

Where both the bulbar and palpebral surfaces of the conjunctiva have full-thickness burns, care needs to be taken to prevent adhesions forming. Treatment by daily rodding using a glass rod is both painful and traumatic; the burnt surfaces should be kept apart with a contact lens that fits into the fornices.

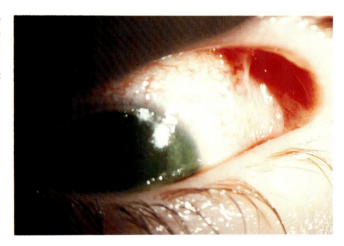

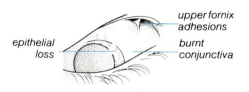

Fig.4.17 Fornix adhesions developing after a lime burn.

The Walser shell (a large contact lens with a central gap corresponding to the cornea) is very effective in keeping the burnt surfaces apart, but may cause pressure on an ischaemic limbus if badly fitted. A large bandage soft contact lens extending into the fornices can also be used, but is not always successful in preventing symblepharon.

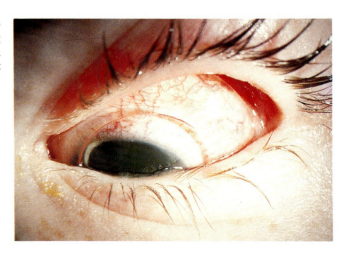

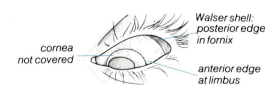

Fig.4.18 Walser shell in position.

Attention should be directed to the prevention of punctal obliteration in burns involving the medial canthus; if identifiable, burnt punctae should be dilated twice daily after instilling anaesthetic drops.

Lid margin burns are treated conservatively initially; if necrosis extends into the lower fornix (as may occur in some molten metal burns), early conjunctival grafting should be performed to help reduce fibrosis leading to entropion. The management of extensive fornix and eyelid burns is discussed later (page 4.15).

Summary of Treatment

All Burns

Emergency irrigation of chemical burns.
Debridement of necrotic tissues.
Analgesia.
Topical antibiotics and mydriatics.
Firm eye pad.

Measures to prevent symblepharon.
Anti-glaucoma treatment if required.

Regular conjunctival cultures to detect bacterial colonisation.

Severe Grade III & IV Burns

If progressive alkali,
    Subconjunctival heparinised blood.
    Consider paracentesis and intracameral lavage.
    Emergency corneal grafting.

All severe burns,
    10% ascorbate drops.
    0.5% disodium edetate if epithelialisation stops.
    Bandage soft contact lens for persisting epithelial defects.
    Early corneal grafting for liquefactive necrosis.

If bilateral,
    Consider cyclophosphamide treatment.

The Results of Healing and Subsequent Treatment

Cornea

Following a corneal burn, epithelial loss is repaired by regeneration from the undamaged margin and occurs quickly if there is no underlying stromal involvement. If Bowman's layer has been affected, epithelialisation will be considerably retarded, often taking two or more weeks to complete.

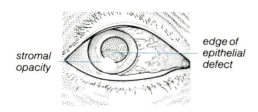

stromal opacity — edge of epithelial defect

Fig.4.19 Caustic soda burn at one week (see Fig. 4.6).

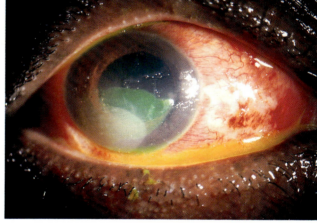

Mild stromal involvement may resolve, but more severe damage leads to thinning and irregularity of the surface, with fibrovascular ingrowth and scarring (see Fig.4.22). These changes reach a peak about two months after injury, then slowly improve. The final degree of opacity and irregularity cannot be judged until at least twelve months after injury.

Some chemical mixtures may cause precipitation within the stroma resulting in a permanent deposit.

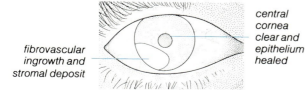

fibrovascular ingrowth and stromal deposit — central cornea clear and epithelium healed

    Fig.4.20 Appearance of the above injury at three months.

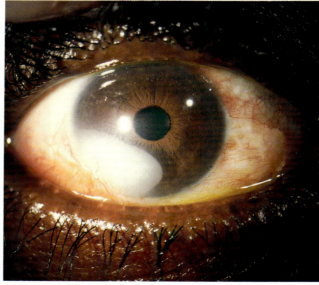

If the changes are axial, vision will be severely reduced, but even peripheral scarring may lead to irregular astigmatism which is optically difficult to correct. The scarring and surface irregularity also result in considerable disability by scattering light and causing glare.

In corneal burns adjacent to the limbus, conjunctival tissues may become hyperplastic and extend onto the burnt surface causing a pseudopterygium.

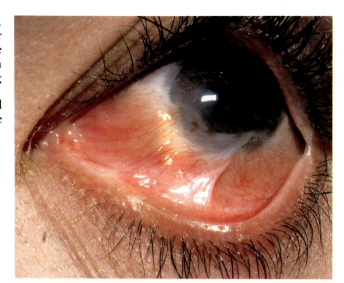

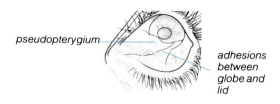

Fig. 4.21 Corneal scarring and pseudopterygium.

If the damage has been severe enough to lead to necrosis and perforation, and early keratoplasty has not been performed, iris tissue may prolapse and plug the leak; this provides an additional source of vascular ingrowth and forms a very dense scar (adherent leukoma). All Grade III and IV burns will lead to a vascularised opaque cornea.

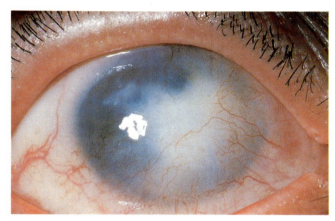

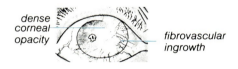

Fig. 4.22 Severely scarred cornea after an ammonia burn. By courtesy of Mr. T.A. Casey.

Damaged endothelium does not recover, and in full-thickness burns the denuded Descemet's membrane is repopulated by fibroblast-like cells; these proliferate to form a retrocorneal membrane.

Treatment of corneal scarring
The disability from glare and astigmatism can be reduced with appropriate spectacles or contact lenses, but axial scarring may need reconstructive surgery to restore vision. Careful assessment is necessary before this is planned: deep corneal vascularisation is common after burns, and in this situation penetrating keratoplasty carries a high risk of rejection.

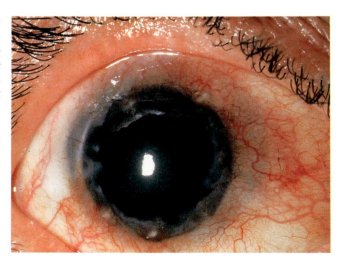

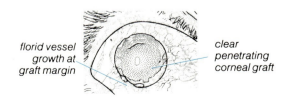

Fig. 4.23 Penetrating corneal graft attracting new vessels. By courtesy of Mr. T.A. Casey.

With penetrating keratoplasty, a technique combining conjunctival recession back to the rectus muscle insertions with a 7.5 mm corneal graft (retaining the donor epithelium), using soft contact lenses and collagenase inhibitors in the postoperative period, has a 50% chance of success. A preliminary lamellar graft may help to reduce the vascularisation and to provide thickness to the cornea.

If this fails, a keratoprosthesis may be the only solution (for the technique see page 8.4); in general, no reconstructive surgery should be attempted except in desperate cases, where the eye is anaesthetic and devoid of lacrimal secretion, or has a poorly controlled glaucoma.

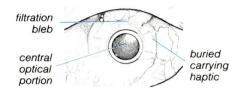

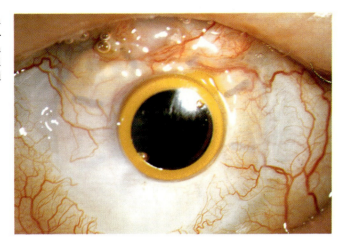

Fig. 4.24   Keratoprosthesis in the only eye after facial burns.

Conjunctiva

The superficial injuries accompanied by chemosis and epithelial loss heal without scarring, although a disturbance of the tear film may result from damage to the goblet cells of the conjunctiva. The deeper burns with ischaemia and necrosis of the episcleral tissues heal by granulation from adjacent unaffected tissues. If localised, no subsequent treatment is required.

If ischaemic damage affects the conjunctival fornices or opposing surfaces of the conjunctiva, contractures and adhesions will develop, resulting in distortion of the lid margin or tethering of the globe (see Fig. 4.21). Damage to the upper fornix may occlude the lacrimal gland ductules, leading to impaired tear secretion. Localised tethering or obliteration of the fornices may not require any active treatment; irritation from disturbed tear formation is common, and will require replacement therapy.

More extensive involvement is often accompanied by damage to the tarsal plate and lid margin, with cicatricial entropion. Its management is discussed in Chapter 10 (see page 10.4).

Sclera and underlying structures

Full-thickness scleral burns will lead to liquefaction and necrosis, resulting in a staphyloma: the underlying uveal tract is visible in the defect as a bulging dark area, with the pupil displaced towards it. The staphyloma usually becomes covered by conjunctiva, and providing the intraocular pressure is controlled, further treatment is not required.

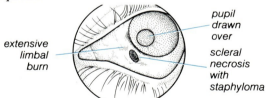

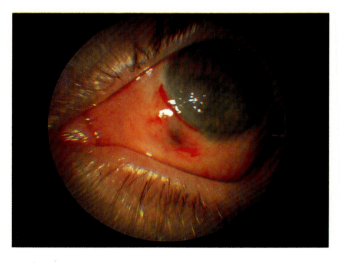

Fig. 4.25   Scleral staphyloma following a full-thickness burn. By courtesy of Mr. S.S.F. Munro.

Extensive limbal involvement with damage to the ciliary body and trabecular meshwork leads to a protracted period of uveitis and an unstable intraocular pressure. This may settle with medical treatment, but damage to the trabecular meshwork (both from direct injury and from peripheral anterior synechiae) may lead to chronic glaucoma.

This can be an intractable problem; medical treatment is tried first, using the full range of preparations available. If this fails to control the intraocular pressure, surgery must be considered. If extensive conjunctival damage is present, drainage surgery is unlikely to be successful, and cyclotherapy is indicated.

Lens

In severe injuries with anterior segment ischaemia, cataract formation is likely. This may rapidly become mature with shallowing of the anterior chamber, and may necessitate surgical intervention. Where possible this should be performed through as small an incision as possible, using a microsurgical cutter to perform a lensectomy, using a bimanual technique.

If the cataract develops slowly and is accompanied by corneal scarring that requires grafting, the extraction can be carried out when corneal surgery is undertaken. These techniques are discussed in detail in Chapter 8.

Chemical burns causing severe facial injury are uncommon, but may occur from attempted assassination with concentrated sulphuric acid or from industrial accidents. A severe ocular burn is more likely than in thermal injuries.

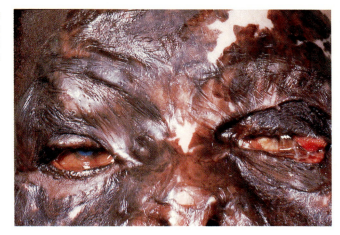

Fig. 4.26   Face and eye burns from concentrated sulphuric acid. By courtesy of Mr. T.A. Casey.

Thermal burns affecting the face and eyes can be part of a widespread injury or can be localised to the face from a fall into an open fire during a period of transient loss of consciousness. The latter are unlikely to have extensive burns that threaten life, but the severe destruction of the facial tissues creates multiple problems.

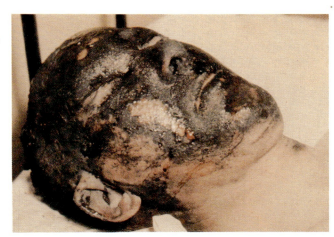

Fig.4.27   Facial burns on presentation.   By courtesy of Mr. D. Jackson.

In this type of burn the reflex lid closure together with Bell's phenomenon often protects the eyes from any major injury, but the eyelids may be affected.   The depth of burn is difficult to judge on presentation, but by ten days the extent of any full-thickness damage will be evident.

Although the globe may be undamaged, if the facial burns are full-thickness with eyelid involvement, subsequent exposure or infection will put the eye at risk.

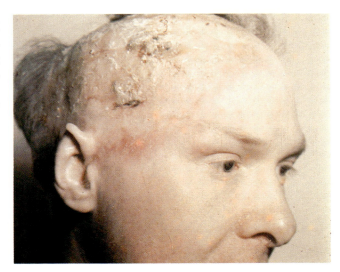

Fig.4.28   Appearance of the above injury nine days later.   By courtesy of Mr. D. Jackson.

The Assessment and Treatment of Facial and   Eyelid Burns

Failure to appreciate the severity of burns involving the eyelid tissues can result in defective treatment, leading to serious deformity and blindness from the complication of exposure.

Skin burns are graded according to the extent and depth of involvement: superficial burns show erythema and oedema only, while partial-thickness burns produce blistering and exudation; marked tissue swelling develops within 24 hours of injury. Full-thickness skin burns show surface coagulation and necrosis; cutaneous sensation is lost, and the absence of pain is a bad sign. As already indicated, the extent of full-thickness involvement cannot be determined at the outset, therefore a policy of waiting for demarcation is adopted.

Prevention of infection

With extensive facial burns which may be a mixture of partial and full-thickness injury, exudation is a prominent feature and encourages bacterial colonisation; a policy of exposure and drying is usually adopted with the application of betadine solution to the affected areas. Alternatively, burnt areas on the face can be covered with tulle gras and sealed with medical silastic foam; this normally remains in position for up to ten days but can be peeled off earlier if required. It is resistant to colonisation by bacteria and helps reduce the risk of infection and contractures.

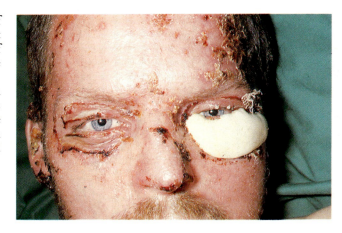

Fig. 4.29 Silastic foam used to protect skin burns or grafts. By courtesy of Mr. A.R. Groves.

The early detection of infection is important in these injuries; the necrotic tissue and exudate provides an environment that microbial growth thrives on, and repeated cultures both of the burnt area and of the conjunctiva should be taken to detect colonisation. This takes place before clinical infection is apparent and positive conjunctival cultures are usually found by the fifth day after a facial burn. There is evidence to suggest that prophylactic ophthalmic treatment with some antibiotic combinations may favour colonisation by more virulent Gram-negative bacteria. Initially, therefore, simple ocular lubricants should be used where necessary, changing to vigorous treatment with appropriate antibiotic drops if colonisation occurs.

Treatment of facial and eyelid burns

Full-thickness skin burns involving the face and eyelids will lead to contracture with ectropion. Children in particular tend to react very quickly to burns, producing excessive fibroplasia in a short period.

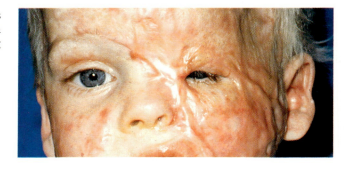

Fig. 4.30 Severe facial burns in a child. By courtesy of Mr. A.R. Groves.

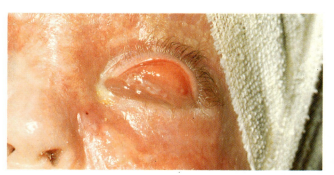

Fig. 4.31 Ectropion developing after seven days. By courtesy of Mr. A.R. Groves.

If ectropion shows signs of developing, early skin grafting is required to prevent exposure. The graft may be protected with silastic foam in a similar way as described above.

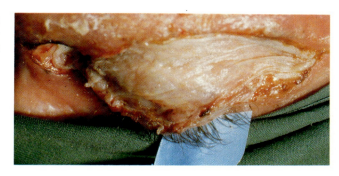

Fig. 4.32 Skin graft applied to correct ectropion. By courtesy of Mr. A.R. Groves.

Burns that destroy the whole eyelid structure are uncommon, but may be seen after an extensive molten metal burn (see Fig. 4.7); the eye has usually suffered severe injury as well. The initial lid swelling protects the eyes from exposure, but within ten days sloughing of the necrotic tissues commences and a severe exposure problem develops.

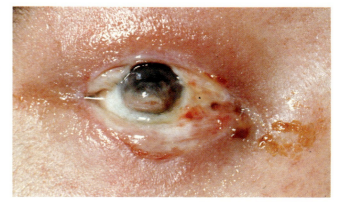

Fig. 4.33 Severe corneal exposure two weeks after a molten metal burn. By courtesy of Mr. J.P. Gowar.

Corneal exposure should be anticipated by early excision of the necrotic tissues with a rotation skin flap lined with mucous membrane to protect the globe.

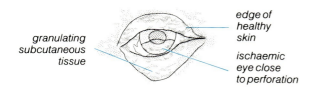

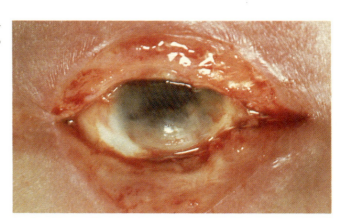

Fig. 4.34 Excision of necrotic lid tissue prior to grafting. By courtesy of Mr. J.P. Gowar.

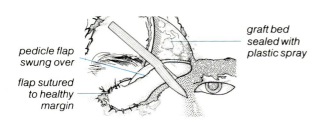

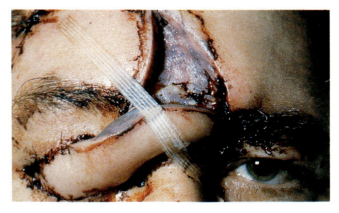

Fig.4.35 A forehead rotation skin flap applied. By courtesy of Mr. J.P. Gowar.

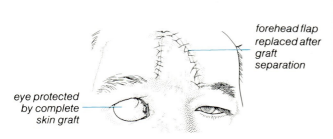

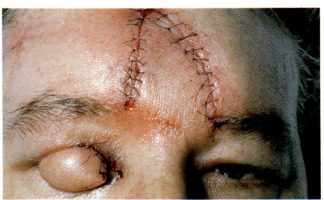

Fig. 4.36 Pedicle divided one month later. By courtesy of Mr. J.P. Gowar.

Any subsequent reconstructive surgery should be deferred for a long period and should take into consideration the extent of the ocular burn and the possibility of reduced tear secretion. An injury of this severity is unlikely to achieve a visual outcome, but preventing exposure and infection allows for the possibility of later treatment, if feasible.

In a less extensive injury, early conjunctival and skin grafting has a better chance of preserving vision. Surgical debridement is carried out after two to three days when demarcation of devitalised tissue has become clear but before exposure and infection have had time to develop. Necrotic tissue is removed first from the skin surface and lid margin back to bleeding points, then the opaque conjunctiva is excised, commencing at the limbus at the junction between healthy and burnt conjunctiva.

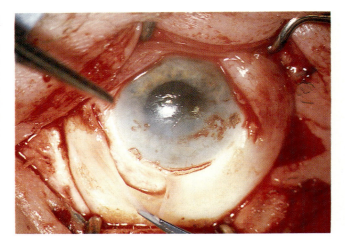

Fig.4.37 Surgical debridement in a grade III molten metal burn (both eyes similarly affected).

The underlying episcleral tissues can then be examined; the integrity of the blood supply to the rectus muscle insertions and the episcleral tissues is a favourable sign. If devitalised as in a grade IV injury, anterior segment ischaemia and ocular perforation are likely (see Fig.4.33). In this instance good episcleral circulation was present.

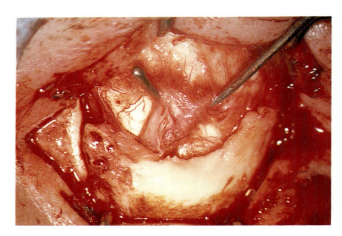

Fig.4.38 Viable inferior rectus muscle identified.

Buccal mucous membrane is taken from the mouth and kept moist until used; if keratoplasty is planned, it should be carried out at this stage. The strip of mucous membrane is then sutured in position, commencing at the lower limbus.

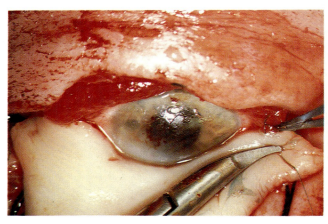

Fig.4.39 Suturing the mucous membrane graft in position.

The lower fornix is formed by several mattress sutures placed deeply in the lid tissues and then brought through the mucous membrane graft. This is then reflected upwards to form the lining of the eyelids, and the free edge is sutured to the viable edge of the conjunctiva above.

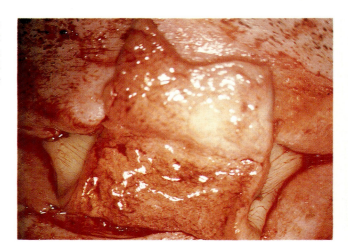

Fig.4.40 Lower fornix formed and mucous membrane graft reflected upwards.

The mucous membrane graft is now lining both the globe and palpebral surfaces; if the upper tarsal plate has been destroyed, nasal septal cartilage is used to replace this.

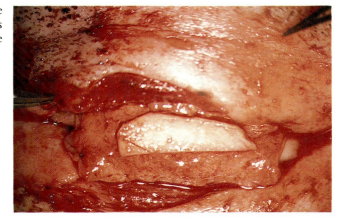

Fig.4.41 Completion of the mucous membrane graft and positioning of nasal septal cartilage.

If still viable, the orbicularis oculi muscle is sutured together over the conjunctival and septal grafts; this provides a vascular bed both for the underlying mucous membrane graft and a free skin graft taken form the retro-auricular region. If the tissues have been extensively devitalised, a pedicle skin flap with its own blood supply is advisable (see Fig.4.35).

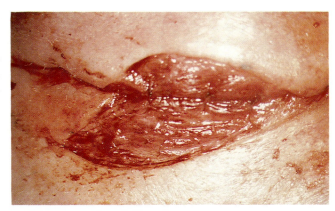

Fig.4.42 Orbicularis muscle repaired prior to applying a free skin graft.

Systemic antibiotics should be given to protect against infection; bacterial cultures and sensitivity should be monitored and therapy changed if indicated. Where possible, the lids should be kept closed for two to three months before opening is carried out.

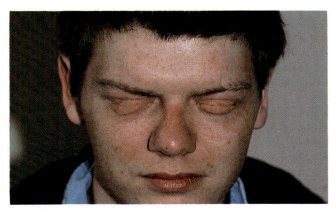

Fig.4.43 Appearance of both eyes before reconstruction three months later.

The tissues are then divided in the natural plane, mobilising the underlying mucous membrane in order to overlap this on the skin surface to allow for retraction of the graft. The presence of good lacrimal secretion is a favourable sign.

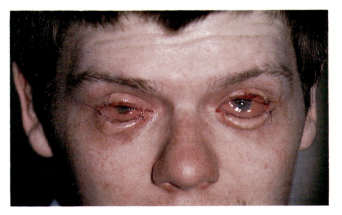

Fig.4.44 Appearance of both eyes eight days after separation.

Early surgery removes devitalised tissue and covers the injured eye so that there is less risk of losing the eye from exposure and infection. Corneal scarring and vascularisation will still occur, but improvement can be expected over several months.

Facial burns

Even if early contracture does not lead to corneal exposure, the progressive cicatrisation of deep facial burns may lead to eventual ectropion of the eyelids, with an unsightly appearance and constant watering of the eyes. Lid retraction may prevent adequate closure and lead to corneal exposure, particularly during sleep.

Cicatricial ectropion after facial burns requires additional skin to be inserted to overcome the contracture (see page 10.4); postauricular or forearm full-thickness skin grafts are used in the eyelid region, as the colour tone matches well.

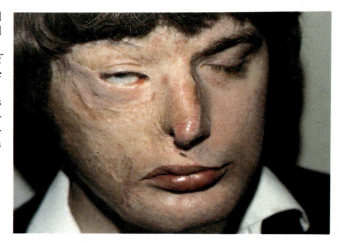

Fig.4.45 Defective lid closure after severe facial burns.

Eyelid burns

The superficial injuries heal without scarring, but the ischaemic injuries heal by granulation and fibrosis; full-thickness lid burns have been described earlier. Localised damage to the lid margin results in destruction of the meibomian orifices, thinning and distortion of the lid margin, and aberrant lash growth.

Obliteration of the tear puncta and canaliculus may occur; in molten metal burns involving the medial canthus, both upper and lower tear ducts may be involved, leading to chronic watering of the eye.

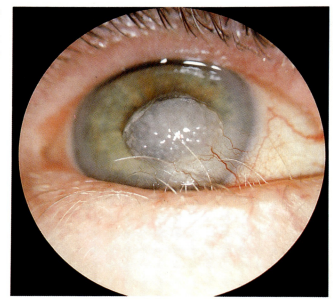

Fig.4.46 Cicatricial entropion with corneal damage.

Treatment of eyelid and associated deformities

The early grafting of conjunctiva or eyelid skin in full-thickness burns reduces the later deformity. If not performed within a week of injury, reconstructive surgery should be delayed until at least six months have elapsed (unless a severe exposure problem develops) to allow the hyperplastic phase of repair to subside. During this period, artificial tear drops or lubricant ointment should be prescribed when necessary, and frequent epilation of aberrant lashes may be required. The surgical management is discussed further in Chapter 10.

APPENDIX

Pharmaceutical preparations

1. Irrigating solution for lime burns (not to be used within 24 hours of injury):
Trisodium edetate injection 5 ml ampoule added to 100 ml of water for injection to give 0.4% solution (0.01 M).

2. Ascorbic acid eye drops:
Ascorbic acid 10%
Potassium bicarbonate 5.7%
Sodium metabisulphite 0.3%
Distilled water to 100%

3. Chelating eye drops:
Disodium edetate 0.25% (0.007 M) and 0.5% (0.013 M) every 2 hours.

The eye drops are prepared without preservative for use in acute burns; the bottles are changed every 24 hours.

5

Blunt Injuries to the Eye

CAUSES OF BLUNT INJURY

A wide variety of injuries can result in ocular contusion: in young adults assault or accidents from sport are the commonest causes; the rise in popularity of squash has led to frequent injury from both racquet and ball. Accidents in the home include injury from elastic luggage straps or champagne corks. Children may be injured when fighting with sticks or stones, or from catapulting paper pellets, while injury from fireworks or air-gun pellets may affect innocent bystanders. In the elderly, a fall onto the edge of a piece of furniture is often the cause; sometimes the force of this injury is sufficient to rupture the globe.

The Pattern of Injury

The site of impact determines the distribution of damage within the eye. In most patients the impact is on the cornea or limbus, causing damage to the underlying vascular tissues. This leads to bleeding into the anterior chamber, and a fluid level of blood is formed. This is known as an *hyphaema*.

After the initial pain accompanying the impact, a dull ache continues for several hours. The vision may be markedly reduced initially, improving as the hyphaema settles.

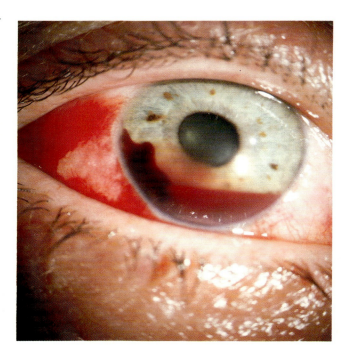

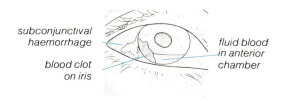

Fig.5.1 Bleeding into the anterior chamber (hyphaema).

Hyphaema is the commonest presentation, but in 10% of patients the impact is over the sclera; there may be no bleeding into the anterior chamber and the brunt of injury is borne by the posterior segment. The eye is comfortable but the patient presents complaining of blurred vision. The fundus appearance ranges from mild retinal oedema to more severe damage. These changes will be described in more detail later (see page 5.12).

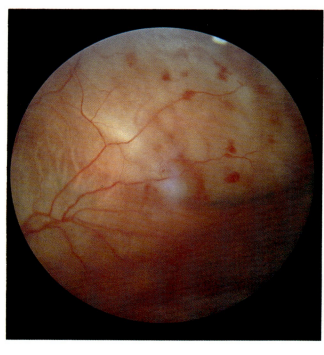

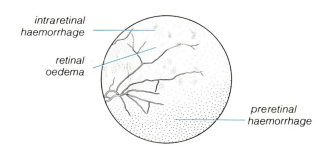

Fig.5.2 Severe retinal oedema following a blunt injury.

Since most of these injuries have an hyphaema, the initial management is concerned with measures to prevent secondary bleeding, and the treatment of this if it occurs.

The full extent of the damage can often only be assessed when the risk of bleeding has passed.

HYPHAEMA

Presentation

With a blunt injury to the eye, the moment of impact is accompanied by intense pain and a sensation of bright light followed by blackness lasting a few seconds; the vision then gradually returns. If the injury has resulted in bleeding into the anterior chamber, there is an abrupt rise of intraocular pressure with continuing pain; the vision remains partly obscured for several hours.

The Initial Assessment of an Hyphaema

1. Note any external evidence indicating the site of impact.

2. Record visual acuity, light projection and pupil reactions.

3. Record extent of hyphaema and source, if visible.

4. Note any anterior segment damage and depth of anterior chamber.

5. Applanation tonometry (NEVER do a digital assessment of pressure).

6. Exclude a ruptured globe.

7. Fundus examination with the direct ophthalmoscope.

8. Check ocular motility.

It is worth making some prediction at this stage of the degree of damage and the anticipated complications: a severe impact with obvious iris or lens damage in addition to the hyphaema carries a higher risk of further bleeding and is more likely to have posterior segment damage.

The Initial Management

In patients with hyphaema the initial management is directed towards preventing secondary bleeding. The incidence of secondary bleeding has been variously reported between 5 - 30%, and the peak incidence is on the second or third day after injury.

Since secondary bleeding may be much more severe than the initial haemorrhage, in-patient treatment is advisable.

Regimen

1. Admit all patients with visible ('macroscopic') hyphaema for strict bed rest for four or more days.

2. Occlude the affected eye with an eye pad.

3. Sedate children to restrict activity if necessary.

4. Treat any corneal abrasion as previously described.

5. Prevent uveitis with prednisolone drops q.i.d.

6. Prevent movement of iris and ciliary body by obtaining full cycloplegia with 1% atropine t.i.d.

There is general agreement that allowing unrestricted activity increases the risk of secondary bleeding; a child with an unrecognised injury may present a day or two later with severe pain from a full secondary hyphaema. Admission to hospital for complete bed rest and observation is advised, although for those with microscopic hyphaemata only, bed rest in the home environment may be acceptable. Clear instructions should be given to return in the event of a sudden recurrence of the pain, and a complete examination is required a week later to exclude any other damage.

Whether it is better to dilate or constrict the pupil or to leave it active has long been a subject of debate. The reported incidence of secondary bleeding varies considerably from one series to another, and no significant difference has emerged between the various regimens. Since the spectrum of injury is so wide, it is difficult to match a treatment group with a control group, or to make a valid comparison between different series. Several studies have supported the concept that secondary bleeding is more common in eyes that have sustained greater damage.

On theoretical grounds, cycloplegia and full mydriasis should immobilise the damaged tissues responsible for the bleeding. This also makes the eye more comfortable and increases the outflow of aqueous via the uveal pathway; this may be important when the drainage angle is clogged with red cells.

The Source of an Hyphaema

Bleeding into the anterior chamber after a blunt injury must arise from either the iris or ciliary body, since these are the vascular tissues in the anterior segment of the eye. The source may be visible, as for example in sphincter tears of the iris or an iridodialysis, where the iris is avulsed from the ciliary body.

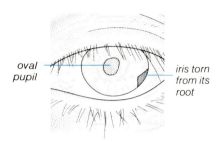

oval pupil — iris torn from its root

Fig.5.3 Iridodialysis.

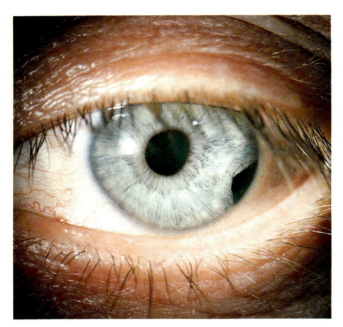

In the majority of patients no visible iris damage is present, and the bleeding has come from a tear into the anterior face of the ciliary body, known as *angle recession*. A trickle of blood may be seen coming from the area of damage, or the site of angle recession may be suspected from a sluggish pupil reaction in the affected quadrant; this may be associated with localised deepening of the anterior chamber. These signs should be recorded, as it may be important to know the origin of the bleeding in the event of a recurrence requiring surgical treatment.

Angle recession can be confirmed later by examining the drainage angle with a gonioscope contact lens, but this should not be done until the risk of secondary bleeding has passed.

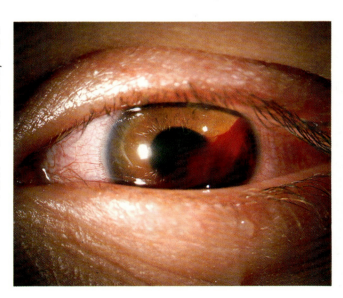

Fig.5.4 Blood tracking down from angle damage.

Hyphaema and the Early Behaviour of Intraocular Pressure

As the bleeding occurs into a confined space there will be an initial rapid rise of intraocular pressure; within a matter of hours this falls to a subnormal level and the acute pain disappears, leaving a mild ache. The intraocular pressure then remains low for several days, particularly in the more severe injuries. Hypotony may persist for several weeks after a severe injury unless complicated by uveitis or secondary bleeding. After recovery of ciliary body function, the intraocular pressure may then swing to high levels and prove difficult to control.

If a patient with a fresh hyphaema presents with a very low intraocular pressure, the possibility of a posterior rupture should be considered; if suspected, the globe should be explored under general anaesthesia. If not recognised at the time of injury, the diagnosis becomes clear when the hyphaema resolves, as the iris/lens diaphragm is retroflexed.

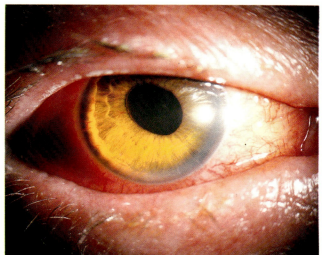

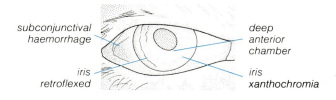

Fig.5.5 Suspected posterior rupture of the globe.

Secondary Hyphaema

Presentation

Secondary bleeding is heralded by the sudden onset of fresh pain in the eye, making the patient restless; this may be short-lived if only a minor bleed occurs. Clot formation generally occurs with a secondary bleed, and the site of the haemorrhage is usually apparent.

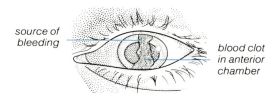

Fig.5.6 Secondary hyphaema with clot formation.

If the bleeding is sufficient to fill the anterior chamber, a vicious circle develops: clot formation causes pupil-block and obstruction to the drainage angle; although aqueous production is low, it is usually sufficient to cause protracted elevation of intraocular pressure. The continuing severe pain makes the patient vomit, and this may precipitate further bleeding. Clot retraction may also contribute, as fresh bleeding tends to occur beneath the existing layer.

The high intraocular pressure and obstruction to aqueous flow causes anoxia, and a full secondary hyphaema assumes a dark appearance: there is marked ciliary injection, loss of corneal transparency from oedema, and the hyphaema appears almost black.

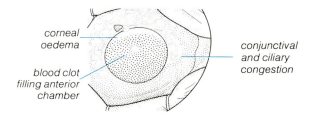

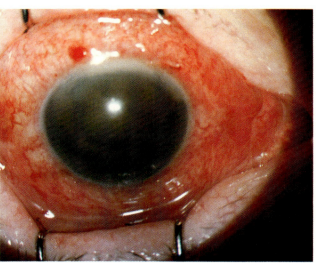

Fig.5.7 Full secondary hyphaema with raised intraocular pressure and corneal oedema.

In mild cases where the secondary haemorrhage has not filled the anterior chamber, the pain and raised pressure rapidly subside and conservative treatment can be continued.

In patients with a full secondary hyphaema the condition must be closely observed, as surgical intervention should be planned after six hours if there is no improvement. Acetazolamide 500mg is given by slow intravenous injection, together with intramuscular injection of an anti-emetic and an analgesic. Intravenous mannitol (1.5g/kg) can be given instead and may be more effective, but is best reserved for immediate pre-operative use.

If the patient is not already receiving mydriatic drops, atropine 1% should be instilled at this stage. This may help overcome the pupil block from the clot, contributing to pain relief.

Continuing pain and restlessness indicate no response to treatment; the cornea remains oedematous, and the dark appearance of the hyphaema persists. Relief of pain and clearing of the cornea indicate improvement; if there is doubt about this, the intraocular pressure is checked by applanation. *Digital assessment of pressure should never be performed.*

The dangers of leaving a secondary hyphaema with raised intraocular pressure are blood-staining of the cornea (from breakdown products of haemoglobin entering a decompensated cornea) and gross iris atrophy with loss of pigment and sphincter damage. If left too long, the raised pressure may compromise the circulation of the optic disc, resulting in permanent visual loss from ischaemic optic neuropathy. All these changes are largely irreversible, although the blood-staining of the cornea may improve with time.

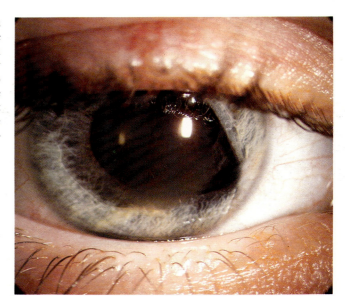

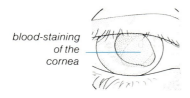

blood-staining of the cornea

Fig. 5.8 Blood-staining of the cornea after a secondary hyphaema.

Surgical Treatment

If after six hours there has been no improvement, surgery should be planned. The aim of surgery is to break the vicious circle by overcoming the pupil block; the site of bleeding should not be disturbed.

The patient is given intravenous mannitol (1.5g/kg) just before surgery to try to reduce the intraocular pressure before opening the eye; continuous positive pressure ventilation may also help reduce the pressure during anaesthesia. A small corneal incision is made, and the anterior chamber adjacent to the wound is gently irrigated with a balanced salt solution. A peripheral iridectomy is then performed and the wound closed with 10.0 monofilament nylon. The bulk of the clot is *not disturbed* as this may precipitate further bleeding. At the end of the procedure a subconjunctival injection of betamethasone 4 mg is given, plus topical antibiotics and 1% atropine.

Occasionally fresh bleeding commences during surgery, and the anterior chamber may refill with blood; if this occurs, it is best to wait five minutes and attempt a further gentle washout of the anterior chamber before closing the wound. Sometimes a bleeding point may be accessible to direct cautery using an intraocular probe attached to the bipolar wet-field cautery (see Fig.7.19).

Analgesics and anti-emetics are important to avoid restlessness in the postoperative period, and strict bed rest must be maintained for a further three to four days to prevent recurrence. A topical steroid/antibiotic combination and 1% atropine drops are prescribed for uveitis.

The success of this simple procedure depends on overcoming pupil block by performing a peripheral iridectomy; recurrent secondary bleeding in the post-operative period may be a problem, and repeat surgery is occasionally required.

Fibrinolytic agents have been recommended in the surgical management of this condition; there is however no particular advantage in attempting to remove all the clot, and as the corneal endothelium is already compromised, the introduction of potentially damaging fluids into the anterior chamber should be kept to a minimum.

An alternative approach (if available) is to use a controlled suction/cutting device (e.g. Ocutome) via two small corneal incisions; a bimanual technique with a separate infusion line on a blunt 20-gauge needle is used. In a full hyphaema with corneal oedema this must be a blind procedure, and complications such as lens damage may occur. As it is unnecessary to remove the bulk of the clot, this procedure is not recommended.

OTHER INTRAOCULAR DAMAGE

In the majority of patients with an hyphaema the risk of secondary bleeding has passed by the fifth day, and the patient can then be mobilised. A full ocular examination is performed to assess the extent of damage; this should include slit-lamp examination and gonioscopy to examine the drainage angle, followed by full pupil dilation for fundus examination, using the indirect ophthalmoscope to examine the peripheral retina.

ANTERIOR SEGMENT DAMAGE

Iris Damage

A mild concussion injury may simply cause scattering of pigment cells from the pigment epithelium of the iris; these may form an imprint of the pupil margin on the surface of the lens (*Vossius' ring*). Pigment cells in the anterior chamber must be distinguished from a microscopic hyphaema; with the magnification of the slit-lamp, red cells have a small uniform appearance, while the pigment cells are larger and more irregular.

After a more severe impact, *radial splits* affecting the pigment epithelium of the iris may be visible with retro–illumination, and *sphincter tears* of the pupil margin may be present.

The above changes follow a central corneal impact, whereas a limbal impact can disrupt the iris root causing an *iridodialysis* (see Fig.5.3).

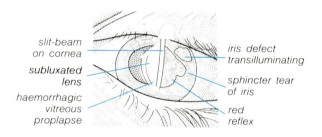

slit-beam on cornea — iris defect transilluminating
subluxated lens — sphincter tear of iris
haemorrhagic vitreous proplapse — red reflex

Fig.5.9 Radial splits and sphincter tear of the iris.

Any of these tears of the iris indicates significant impact on the eye, and other damage is likely to be present. Lens damage is a common association, but posterior segment damage must also be suspected.

An iridodialysis is always a sign of severe limbal impact, and recurrent secondary bleeding is common; patients with this injury should not be mobilised too early.

When the risk of secondary bleeding has passed, these patients should be carefully examined with the indirect ophthalmoscope, as a retinal dialysis is a common association.

If tears of the sphincter margin are present, pupil dilation should be avoided; it is better to leave the pupil mobile, otherwise posterior synechiae to the lens may occur. One or two sphincter tears will have little effect on pupil function, but several tears in association with pigment epithelial splits often result in a dilated atonic pupil. This may lead to photophobia and reduced vision, and the patient may subsequently require tinted glasses.

A large iridodialysis may cause dazzle and monocular diplopia, particularly if the defect is situated laterally or inferiorly. The symptoms may be sufficiently trouble-some to merit reconstruction at a later date; however, at least one year should elapse before surgery is under-taken, unless lens damage makes earlier intervention necessary (for the surgical technique see page 8.14).

Angle Recession

This term is used to describe tears into the anterior face of the ciliary body, which alter the appearance of the drainage angle. This type of damage is found in almost all patients who have had a visible hyphaema.

The drainage angle of the anterior chamber can only be examined using a contact lens with an angled mirror (gonioscope) and the slit-lamp microscope. When gonioscopy is performed, it is helpful to compare the injured eye with the healthy one; in this way it is easier to recognise the subtle changes in the angle appearance.

Shallow tears consist of separation of the uveal processes, so that the scleral spur and ciliary body band become more easily visible.

Moderate tears are characterised by a definite cleft into the face of the ciliary body between the circular and longitudinal muscle fibres; the angle appears wider and deeper than that of the normal eye.

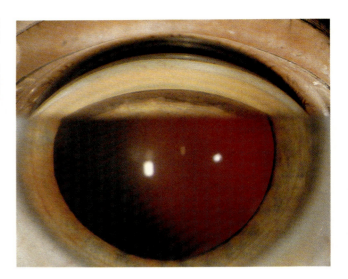

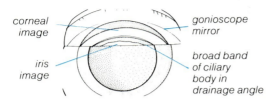

Fig.5.10 Moderate angle recession seen with the gonioscope lens.

In *severe tears* the apex of the cleft cannot be visualised.

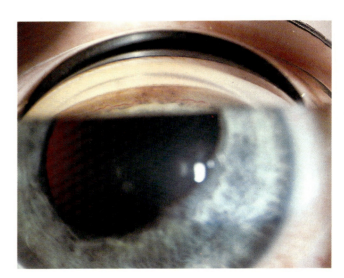

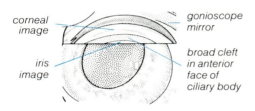

Fig.5.11 Deep angle recession exposing the major arterial circle.

The site of these deeper angle recessions may be suspected from atonicity of the pupil in the affected quadrant.

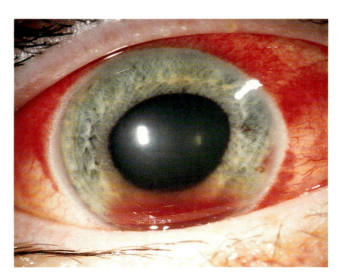

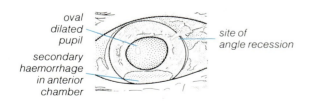

Fig.5.12 Traumatic mydriasis with secondary hyphaema; angle recession in the affected quadrant.

Extensive angle recession may be associated with traumatic mydriasis which persists for several months; this is associated with poor accommodation and difficulty with reading.

Shallow tears are less extensive than the deeper clefts, and rarely extend into more than one quadrant; they become more difficult to recognise with time, and are unlikely to lead to late glaucoma. In 50% of patients with an hyphaema, a shallow angle recession of less than 90° is the only damage sustained.

Moderate and deep tears are often more extensive, and are associated with permanent damage to the outflow pathways. In the long run this leads to atrophy and replacement fibrosis of the affected trabecular meshwork, which may lead to unilateral glaucoma many years after the initial injury.

Late glaucoma has only been reported when the angle recession exceeds 180°; the risk increases if the tear exceeds 240°. These extensive tears are uncommon, affecting only 15% of contusion injuries; in these patients there is a strong correlation with other anterior segment damage, particularly with lens subluxation, and the initial hyphaema often persists for more than 24 hours. Annual follow-up is recommended for patients with angle recession exceeding 180° to watch for the late development of glaucoma.

The cause of angle recession

There is a clinical correlation between the site of impact and the extent and distribution of the angle recession: a central corneal impact often results in extensive angle recession and lens subluxation; after a limbal impact (which is often associated with localised lens opacities) the apex of the angle recession is at this point, while an impact behind the limbus gives angle recession in the opposite quadrant (see Figs.5.27–5.29). This suggests that lens displacement with traction on the ciliary body via the zonule is the cause of angle recession.

Experimental studies have shown that a central corneal impact deforms the globe and causes a posterior movement of the lens at a time when the anterior sclera is expanding. The cornea and anterior sclera recover rapidly from deformation but the displaced lens has a greater inertia which leads to a shearing force between the lens and the ciliary body, resulting in tears into the anterior face and, in severe cases, rupture of the zonule with lens dislocation.

A similar shearing force may also develop between the lens and the vitreous base, particularly after a limbal impact when the lens may be tilted; this may lead to avulsion of the vitreous base and retinal dialysis.

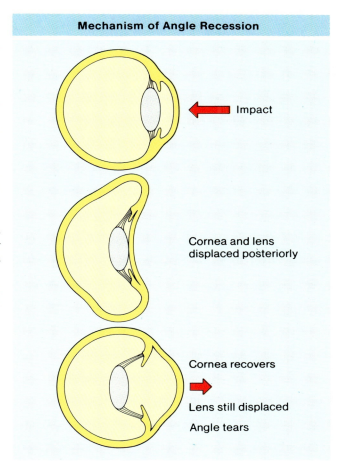

Mechanism of Angle Recession

← Impact

Cornea and lens displaced posteriorly

Cornea recovers

Lens still displaced

Angle tears

Fig.5.13 Diagram showing distortion of the globe after a corneal impact.

Lens Damage

The lens may be displaced from its normal position by rupture of the zonule, or it may suffer structural damage resulting in opacification or even rupture.

Changes in lens position

The mechanism of lens subluxation or dislocation has already been described above; the whole zonule is rarely disrupted (except in an elderly person or in patients with a congenital weakness of the zonule), but the lens may be tilted, with herniation of the vitreous gel through the pupil (see also Fig.5.9).

Minor degrees of lens subluxation require no immediate surgical treatment, but uveitis and progressive cataract formation are common. Accomodative failure and astigmatism will require spectacle correction.

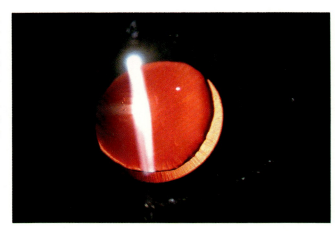

Fig.5.14 Lens subluxation seen against the red reflex.

Extensive disruption of the zonule leads to instability of the lens; subluxation into the anterior chamber may occur, causing a rapid rise of intraocular pressure from a pupil block glaucoma. Similarly, a forward movement of the lens behind the iris may lead to shallowing of the anterior chamber and a rise of intraocular pressure from angle closure. This rarely develops during the first week after injury because of hypotony from impaired ciliary body function; when this recovers the patient develops severe supraorbital pain, injection and corneal oedema from raised intraocular pressure.

Initially the raised intraocular pressure is controlled by a slow intravenous injection of acetazolamide 500 mg, and the pupil is dilated with 1% atropine drops. Topical steroids are given to control uveitis and the patient is positioned supine to allow the lens to settle back. Once the intraocular pressure is controlled, the position and stability of the lens can be assessed.

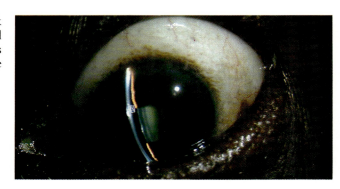

If the lens is behind the pupil but causing a pupil block because of forward movement, an elective peripheral iridectomy is performed. This is preferable to a lens extraction at this stage, as it is a smaller procedure, and the subluxated lens may remain clear.

Fig.5.15 Shallowing of the anterior chamber after traumatic lens subluxation (slit-view).

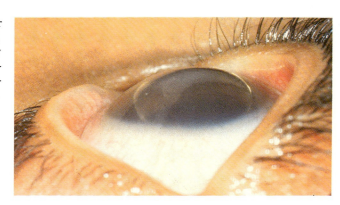

If, however, the lens is subluxating into the anterior chamber and cannot be repositioned behind the pupil, lens extraction or lensectomy will be required. This may need to be performed as an emergency if medical treatment fails to bring down the intraocular pressure; preoperative mannitol 1.5 g/kg is given just prior to surgery.

Fig.5.16 A clear lens dislocated into the anterior chamber.

A posterior subluxation or dislocation is treated conservatively initially, but visual problems or uveitis may necessitate surgery. The techniques for all these problems are discussed in Chapter 8 (see pages 8.8–10).

Structural lens damage

Mild concussion leads to small white opacities on the anterior surface of the lens. These are sometimes reversible, but more often they persist as small opacities which become buried beneath clear cortex.

After more severe concussion, cortical lens opacities develop. A posterior rosette opacity developing within hours of injury is likely to progress to cataract formation, although in young children such changes may be reversible.

Localised peripheral lens opacities may remain static for some time, but ultimately lead to a progressive cataract. This is a common complication associated with an iridodialysis.

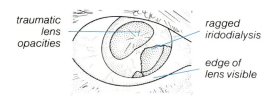

traumatic lens opacities

ragged iridodialysis

edge of lens visible

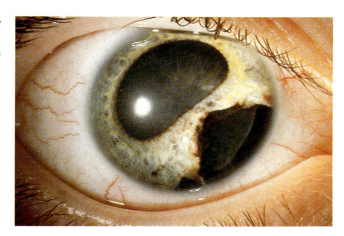

　Fig.5.17 Progressive cataract associated with iridodialysis.

The lens capsule may be ruptured at the time of injury and this is likely to lead to rapid swelling of the lens with flocculation of soft lens matter into the anterior chamber, uveitis, and possibly angle closure glaucoma.

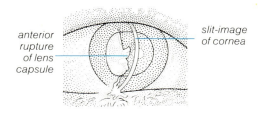

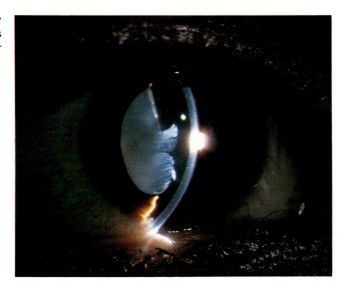

anterior rupture of lens capsule

slit-image of cornea

Fig.5.18 Lens rupture following blunt injury.

The surgical management of a traumatic cataract can usually be deferred unless capsule rupture has occurred. In general it is preferable to delay surgery for at least six months, as macular damage often coexists and there is an increased risk of postoperative cystoid macular oedema. Early surgical intervention will, however, be required if the capsule has ruptured; the techniques involved are discussed in Chapter 8 (see pages 8.5-7).

Uveitis and Raised Intraocular Pressure

A mild degree of uveitis accompanies all contusion injuries, but in some situations it is severe and persistent. Any patient with a pre-existing history of uveitis may have an unusually severe reaction to injury, and this should be anticipated.

As described earlier, the intraocular pressure is usually low during the first week after injury (with the exception of secondary bleeding), but when ciliary body function recovers, the intraocular pressure may swing to high levels.

Causes of protracted uveitis and raised intraocular pressure

1. Secondary hyphaema.

2. Lens rupture or rapid cataract formation.

3. Lens subluxation with pupil-block glaucoma.

4. Posterior dislocation of the lens.

5. Dense vitreous haemorrhage.

Patients who have required surgical treatment for secondary bleeding often have a persisting uveitis for some weeks, which generally responds to topical steroids. Uveitis and raised intraocular pressure may complicate certain types of lens damage; surgical treatment is often required, as discussed earlier (see page 5.10).

The most intractable cases of persisting uveitis and raised intraocular pressure are associated with *vitreous haemorrhage*. These patients have had a severe injury with posterior segment damage; lens subluxation and extensive angle recession are often present as well. After an initial period of hypotony which may last several weeks, a severe glaucoma may develop that can be extremely difficult to control. The medical regimen includes the use of atropine, and adrenergic or beta-blocking drops together with oral medication with acetazolamide tablets 250 mg q.i.d. and potassium supplements. Pilocarpine drops are not very helpful and increase discomfort in an inflamed eye. Anti-inflammatory drops will be required if the uveitis is severe.

Even with full medical treatment, the intraocular pressure may remain very high and surgical treatment has to be considered. It is often difficult to be certain whether the raised pressure is due principally to uveitis, lens damage, or red cell fragments reaching the anterior chamber and clogging up a compromised drainage angle. A steroid-induced rise of pressure must also be considered. Drainage surgery is often unsuccessful in the presence of uveitis, and vitrectomy with or without lensectomy may need to be considered. This problem is further discussed in the next section on posterior segment damage (see page 5.18).

5.11

Injury to the posterior segment can result from an impact over the sclera, leading to direct mechanical damage to the underlying choroid and retina. Both this and a more anterior impact also cause severe distortion of the globe and transmission of shock waves; these factors contribute to damage remote from the site of impact. Any injury can therefore be associated with damage to the structures at the posterior pole of the eye, or to the peripheral retina and choroid. Although both types of damage may coexist, it is convenient to discuss them separately.

Damage to the Posterior Pole of the Eye

Of all the patients with an hyphaema, 30% are subsequently found to have some damage to the posterior pole of the eye. The changes range from mild macular oedema to severe oedema with intraretinal haemorrhages; chorioretinal ruptures may also occur with subretinal haemorrhage. The severity of visual impairment depends on whether the fovea is directly involved. The worst damage follows an evulsion of the optic nerve, which usually leads to total loss of vision.

Macular oedema

This corresponds to peripheral 'commotio retinae' and represents cloudy swelling of the retina, with impairment of function. The macular region loses its transparency and the foveal reflex is lost. In many contusion injuries, the posterior segment may not be visible for one or two days, and mild macular oedema may recover in this period. Oedema that persists beyond five days reflects more than a temporary concussion effect on axonal transport, and indicates a disturbance of the retinal capillary circulation. In the more severe cases small intraretinal haemorrhages occur, and the reduction in vision may be profound.

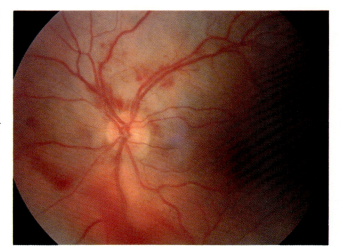

Fig.5.19 Severe traumatic oedema with intraretinal haemorrhage (see also Fig.5.2).

In mild cases complete resolution may occur, but in most patients where the oedema persists for more than a few days *pigment scarring* of the retina will develop as the oedema clears. If the fovea itself is spared, visual recovery may be quite good.

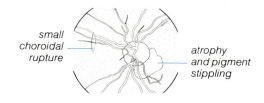

small choroidal rupture

atrophy and pigment stippling

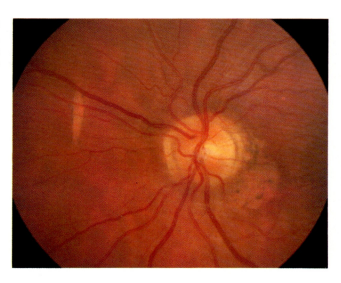

Fig.5.20 Pigment scarring adjacent to optic disc. (Note small choroidal rupture on nasal side).

Management
There is no specific treatment for this condition, but on general principles rest during the first few days is advisable, with protection against light damage using dark glasses. Frequent examination with the indirect ophthalmoscope or fundus camera should be avoided for the same reason.

Macular damage may occur in conjunction with a peripheral retinal injury, but is most often found after a central corneal impact; it is common in those patients who eventually develop a progressive cataract. This is a point to bear in mind when considering surgery for a traumatic cataract.

In the more severe forms of oedema, recovery may be quite slow and visual function continues to improve over six months or more. In some patients an initial improvement may be followed by a sudden deterioration which indicates the development of cystic degeneration leading to a macular hole; this will result in permanent impairment of vision.

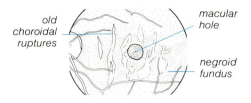

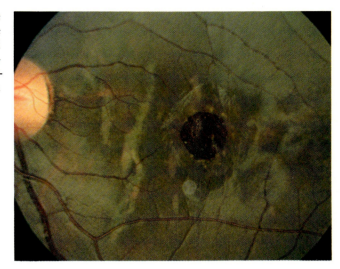

Fig.5.21 Macular hole after severe macular oedema (choroidal ruptures are also present).

Choroidal ruptures

This is less common than macular oedema and reflects an injury resulting in considerable distortion of the globe; the stretching of the posterior segment tissues around their fixed attachment to the optic nerve head ruptures the choroid and may disrupt the overlying retina. These ruptures are usually concentric with the optic disc, and may be multiple.

Small ruptures can be present without any major haemorrhage, although some macular oedema usually coexists. In the more extensive ruptures, bleeding from the torn capillaries occurs resulting in a haematoma underneath the retina.

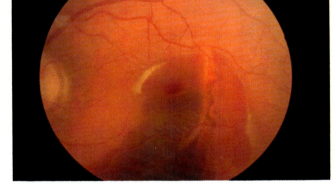

Fig.5.22 Traumatic choroidal haematoma.

Initially the haematoma obscures the underlying choroidal rupture and a large central scotoma is present. The blood will slowly absorb with time, and eventually the rupture becomes visible as a white crescentic streak due to exposure of the underlying sclera (see Figs.5.20 and 5.21).

Slow visual improvement occurs and the visual defect may range from localised scotomata to sector field defects depending on the site of rupture and the extent of the damage.

Management

Any patient with a large choroidal haematoma should be kept on bed rest for several days; the haematoma may rupture through the internal limiting membrane of the retina and result in subhyaloid or vitreous haemorrhage. Absorption of a large choroidal haematoma is likely to take several weeks; generally the risk of vitreous haemorrhage has passed after the first week when mobilisation is commenced. The outcome will not be known until the extent of the underlying damage is revealed.

A late complication of a choroidal rupture is the development of a disciform macular degeneration; this tends to occur with ruptures running close to the fovea. The neovascular complex involves the macula early, and for this reason it is rarely treatable.

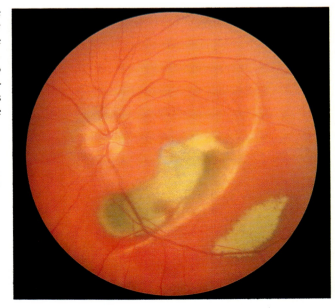

Fig.5.23 A disciform macular scar after a choroidal rupture.

Evulsion of the optic nerve

This devastating complication of a blunt injury may be accompanied by severe damage to the anterior segment, but the latter is often uninvolved in the injury. Optic nerve evulsion either follows a diffuse impact on the globe or injury from a blunt instrument such as a thumb stuck in just above the infraorbital margin; the damage may result from severe compression of the globe against the orbital roof.

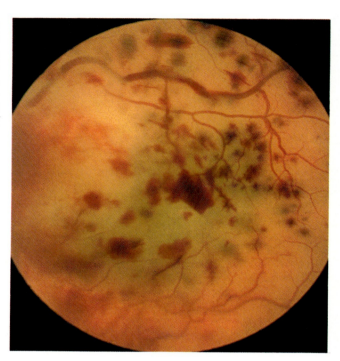

The affected eye presents with blindness, or at best there is some preservation of light perception in the temporal field only; there is a total afferent pupil defect. If seen early, the fundus picture shows signs of widespread retinal infarction, with cloudy swelling of the retina, a cherry-red spot at the macula and florid blot haemorrhages. Preretinal haemorrhage often obscures the optic disc but, if visible, a cleft is seen around the margin of the optic disc at the site of disruption.

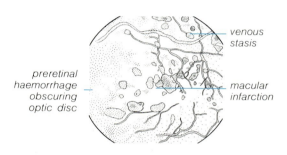

Fig.5.24 Early appearance of an optic nerve evulsion.

Within a matter of hours a major vitreous haemorrhage occurs and obscures any further view. In a few reported cases fluorescein angiography has been possible before vitreous haemorrhage has supervened; this has confirmed the disruption of the retinal circulation and demonstrated massive fluorescein leakage from the cleft at the margin of the optic disc.

There is no visual recovery, although the eye usually retains a good cosmetic appearance. Ultimately a grossly distorted and atrophic optic disc may be visible.

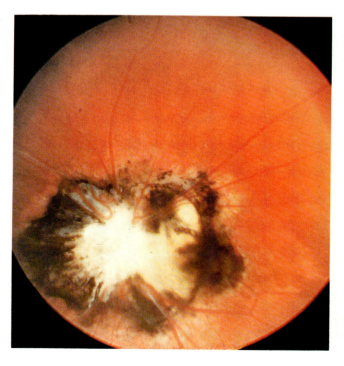

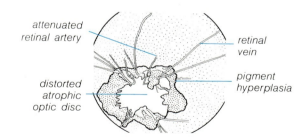

Fig.5.25 Late appearance of an optic nerve evulsion.

It is important to confirm this diagnosis at an early stage, so that the patient can be warned not to expect recovery of vision. In those patients where early vitreous haemorrhage has obscured the view, optic nerve damage can be confirmed by measuring the Visual Evoked Potential: in optic nerve evulsion this will be absent. The electroretinogram will be impaired in the early period after injury, but recovers to normal after some weeks.

Ragged retinal tears

Ragged retinal tears may extend to involve the posterior pole, but these are generally an extension of large peripheral tears and always reflect extensive retinal damage; widespread commotio retinae and haemorrhage may be present. The management of this problem will be discussed in the next section.

Peripheral and Equatorial Retinal or Choroidal Damage

Full dilation of the pupil is required for adequate examination of the peripheral retina; this is performed once the risk of secondary bleeding has passed, usually on the fourth or fifth day after injury. Examination with the indirect ophthalmoscope is required to see right out to the ora serrata, but in a recently contused eye, scleral indentation should be used with caution.

Commotio retinae

Commotio retinae represents a functional derangement of the nerve fibre layer; in mild cases this reflects a temporary disturbance from concussion, while in more severe cases, some disruption of the microcirculation is present with intraretinal haemorrhage. The affected area has a grey translucent appearance and this is always more striking in the negroid fundus. In severe cases a corresponding visual field defect will be present.

Commotio retinae usually reflects direct damage from an impact over the affected retina, and is therefore more common on the temporal side. Mild changes will resolve without trace, but those associated with intraretinal haemorrhage will develop atrophy and pigment scarring in the affected area. Although small atrophic holes may be present with a free operculum, they are not associated with any risk of retinal detachment.

Small haemorrhages into the anterior vitreous base region are a frequent occurrence with severe commotio retinae. These often take a long time to absorb because they are situated in the thick cortical gel; they may obscure a clear view of the peripheral retina for some weeks. They often have a scalloped edge, and may be confused with retinal breaks. These haemorrhages are related to the site of impact representing direct contusion.

Management

Provided there is no anterior segment damage with hyphaema, mild cases of commotio retinae can be allowed home to rest; the more severe injuries (particularly those with intraretinal haemorrhage or those with vitreous haemorrhage obscuring a view of the peripheral retina) should be admitted for bed rest and observation. It is common for small preretinal haemorrhages to break through into the vitreous in the first few days. Unless recurrent vitreous haemorrhage occurs, mobilisation is commenced on the fourth day after injury. Careful follow-up is required, as the full extent of peripheral retinal damage may not be evident until the haemorrhages have cleared.

Major Peripheral and Equatorial Retinal Damage

Of blunt contusion injuries, 10% will have major retinal damage affecting the ora or equator; there are three types of damage, and two of these are associated with a significant risk of retinal detachment. A macroscopic hyphaema is present in only one third of cases, so the initial visual disturbance may be minimal. This reflects a more posterior site of impact in these patients, and they may not present at the time of injury, only seeking advice months or years later when a retinal detachment has occurred.

Types of peripheral retinal damage:

Ragged equatorial retinal tears.
Retinal dialysis at the ora serrata.
Equatorial choroido-retinal ruptures.

Ragged equatorial tears

Irregular tears of the equatorial retina represent a severe degree of disruption from an impact directly over the retina; commonly the injury is caused by a stick or stone that has struck the sclera with considerable force. These tears are always associated with severe surrounding commotio retinae, and the retina may be elevated immediately. Because the surrounding commotio retinae has a tendency to produce pigment scarring, an initial retinal detachment may flatten spontaneously.

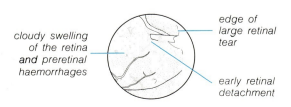

cloudy swelling of the retina *and* preretinal haemorrhages

edge of large retinal tear

early retinal detachment

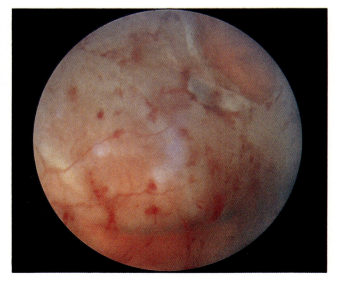

Fig.5.26 Irregular retinal break and commotio retinae.

Management

The relatively good prognosis in these detachments reflects the absence of vitreous traction to these tears. Spontaneous flattening makes the surgical management easier, but cryotherapy around the tear may be required to prevent recurrent detachment. Some patients develop early progressive retinal detachment, and the large irregular size of the tears makes surgical treatment difficult.

Conventional surgery with a radial sponge may be used, but it is often difficult to reach the posterior extent of the tear. In this situation the balloon technique described by Lincoff may be particularly appropriate, as it gives a large smooth indentation that can cover an irregular tear. This technique is described in more detail in Chapter 9 (see page 9.14).

In a severe injury, the tears may be multiple and associated with vitreous haemorrhage and anterior segment damage; severe uveitis is common and surgery is often impracticable.

Retinal dialysis

This usually follows a limbal impact, and is due to shearing forces developing between the lens and vitreous base during the distortion of the globe. The apex of the dialysis is usually related to the site of impact, so direct mechanical disruption plays a part. The retinal dialyses may be multiple, and between the affected bays the vitreous base is often avulsed, suspended like a clothes line, with clumps of pigment epithelium attached.

Although the retrospective studies of Cox, Schepens and Freeman suggested that the upper nasal quadrant is the commonest site for a traumatic retinal dialysis, prospective studies of known trauma at our hospital found the highest incidence in the lower temporal quadrant. This quadrant is the most vulnerable to direct contusion.

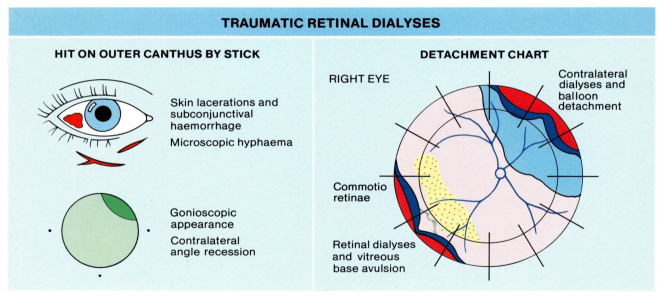

Fig.5.27 Diagram of traumatic retinal dialyses, both at the site of impact in the lower temporal quadrant and via indirect traction on the upper nasal vitreous base.

If a traumatic retinal dialysis is seen within a few days of injury, surrounding commotio retinae is often present, confirming the role of direct trauma. Considerable lifting of the affected retina may be present from the time of injury, but bullous retinal detachment rarely develops until one or two weeks have elapsed. As with the ragged retinal tears, spontaneous flattening of the retinal dialysis may occur during the first two weeks, and this may make the surgical treatment easier.

Management

Although spontaneous flattening with pigment demarcation often occurs, it is advisable to supplement this with two rows of cryotherapy once the eye has settled. Persisting or progressive retinal detachment also requires permanent indentation to seal the retinal break, using a tangential 3 mm sponge.

Provided these retinal dialyses are recognised early, surgical treatment can be expected to have a good outcome. The timing of surgery is judged according to the degree of contusion weighed against the rate of progression of retinal detachment and it is always advisable to wait a few days in the first instance.

In some patients, a very extensive retinal dialysis exceeding 90° reflects a pre-existing weakness; the uninjured eye must also be examined to look for extensive white-without-pressure changes which may carry a risk of giant tear formation. In this situation, prophylactic cryotherapy to the other eye is indicated.

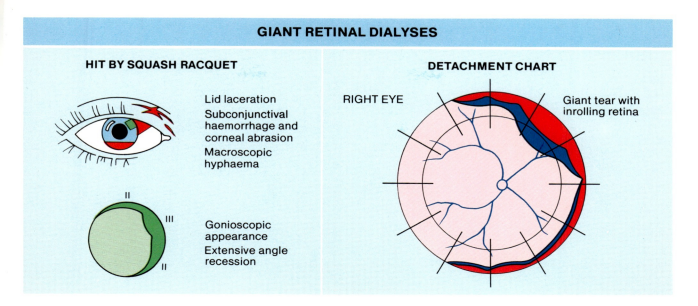

GIANT RETINAL DIALYSES

HIT BY SQUASH RACQUET

Lid laceration

Subconjunctival haemorrhage and corneal abrasion

Macroscopic hyphaema

Gonioscopic appearance

Extensive angle recession

DETACHMENT CHART

RIGHT EYE

Giant tear with inrolling retina

Fig.5.28   Diagram of giant retinal dialysis after blunt injury.

If a dialysis is not recognised at the time of injury, the onset of retinal detachment may be very slow, particularly if the break is below. The progression of retinal detachment is insidious, with partial demarcation and signs of a long duration such as subretinal fibrosis and intraretinal cyst formation. The patient may only present when the subretinal fluid reaches the macula with disturbance of central vision. Despite the long-standing nature of these cases, the prognosis for successful reattachment with surgery is good; the visual outcome will depend on the condition of the macula.

The surgical management of retinal breaks with or without detachment is discussed in more detail in Chapter 9 (see page 9.13).

Choroidal ruptures

This is the third type of peripheral damage seen after a contusion injury, but contrary to the previous examples, the risk of retinal detachment in this case is very low. Peripheral choroidal ruptures occur after a similar injury to that causing ragged equatorial retinal tears, and the two types of damage may coexist.

In general, choroidal ruptures follow a severe localised scleral impact, such as occurs with an air-gun pellet. The ruptures have a different configuration from those occurring at the posterior pole; they are multiple elliptical splits, usually orientated in a radial fashion, accompanied by underlying choroidal haemorrhage and severe commotio retinae. Severe macular oedema is almost invariably present as well.

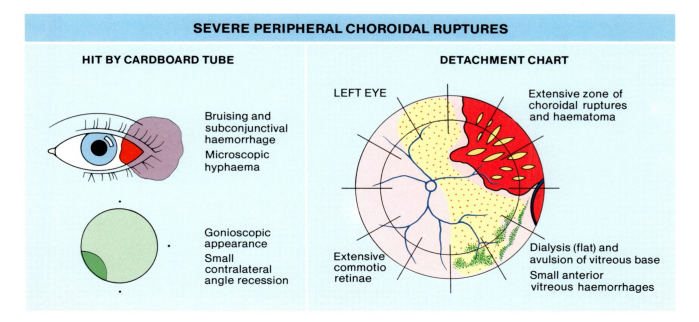

SEVERE PERIPHERAL CHOROIDAL RUPTURES

HIT BY CARDBOARD TUBE

Bruising and subconjunctival haemorrhage

Microscopic hyphaema

Gonioscopic appearance

Small contralateral angle recession

DETACHMENT CHART

LEFT EYE

Extensive zone of choroidal ruptures and haematoma

Extensive commotio retinae

Dialysis (flat) and avulsion of vitreous base

Small anterior vitreous haemorrhages

Fig.5.29   Diagram of severe peripheral choroidal ruptures (small dialysis present as well).

In a very severe injury that is just short of rupturing the globe, both choroid and retina may disintegrate at the site of impact; widespread concussion effects are present.

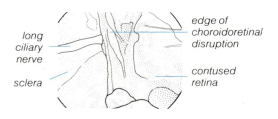

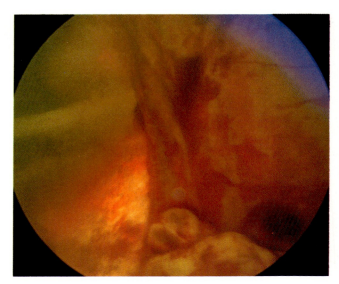

Fig.5.30 Disruption of peripheral retina and choroid after a severe contusion injury.

Despite extensive disruption, retinal detachment is uncommon in these very severe injuries, and healing with gross scarring occurs. Damage to the posterior pole usually coexists.

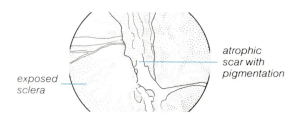

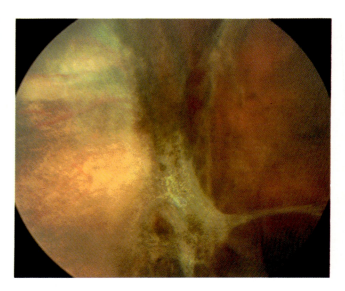

Fig.5.31 Appearance two months later showing gross scarring.

As with posterior choroidal ruptures, there is a risk of vitreous haemorrhage due to a break-through of the underlying choroidal haematoma. In most patients the pigment scarring that develops around these breaks gives firm adhesion between retina and choroid, but very occasionally a retinal detachment will occur if pigment- ation fails to develop.

The management of peripheral choroidal ruptures is identical to those involving the posterior pole, as described earlier (see page 5.13). Only in exceptional cases will any surgical intervention be required.

Other Posterior Segment Problems

Diffuse vitreous haemorrhage

This poses a number of problems: as mentioned earlier, there is often major anterior segment damage, with uveitis and intractable glaucoma; serious posterior segment damage must be present, but while the view is obscured by haemorrhage the development of retinal detachment is difficult to detect. Tests of light projection, electroretinography and ultrasonography help monitor retinal function and position while the view is obscured (see pages 7.2-4).

There is a greater likelihood that the vitreous haemorrhage has come from a break-through of a choroidal haematoma than from a primary retinal tear. Conservative management is followed unless there is clear evidence of retinal detachment. The anterior segment complications are treated along the lines indicated earlier, and even if retinal detachment does occur, the severity of the uveitis and glaucoma may make effective surgical treatment impossible.

Where one suspects that retinal detachment is developing, and the anterior segment problems are controlled, vitreoretinal surgery should be considered. As the eye has suffered a major contusion injury, this should not be undertaken before two weeks have elapsed, as the risks of secondary bleeding during surgery are high during this early period. This is discussed further in Chapter 9 (see page 9.2).

6

Penetrating Eye Injuries

Injuries from a sharp object cause a *laceration* with damage confined to the underlying tissues; the extent ranges from a puncture wound to a laceration transecting the globe. Injury from a blunt object causes contusion and if the force is sufficient it *ruptures* the globe, with widespread damage from internal haemorrhage. These two types of injury are referred to as *perforating eye injuries*, with an open wound and often prolapse of intraocular contents.

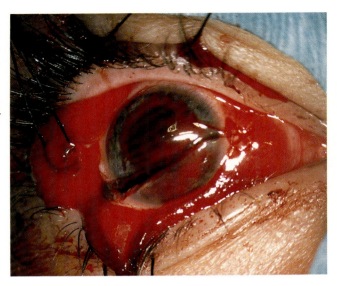

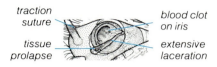

Fig.6.1 Extensive corneoscleral perforation with prolapse of intraocular contents and internal bleeding.

At the other extreme there are injuries due to small metal fragments travelling at speed, which penetrate the eye and cause internal damage; they often have a sealed entry wound with no prolapse. These injuries are commonly referred to as *intraocular foreign bodies*. In addition to mechanical damage, many of these metallic particles, particularly steel or copper, will cause chemical damage if not removed.

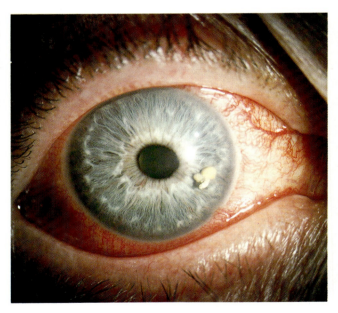

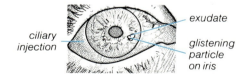

Fig.6.2 Steel foreign body on the iris showing inflammatory reaction.

An overlap between these two groups occurs: 'perforating injuries' may be complicated by a foreign body in the wound, such as glass fragments from a shattered windscreen, while some of the larger 'intraocular foreign bodies' result in an open wound with tissue prolapse. For the typical case, however, the presentation and management of the two problems is very different, so it is helpful to consider the two types of injury separately.

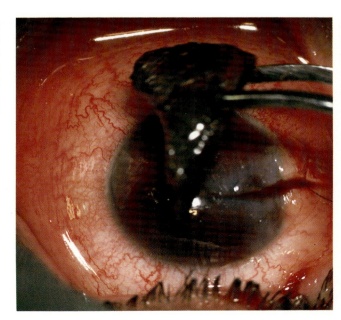

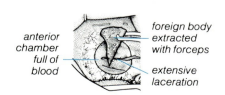

Fig.6.3 'Perforating eye injury' with open wound and tissue prolapse due to a large foreign body.

LACERATIONS AND RUPTURES OF THE GLOBE

The Pattern of Injury

Accidental injury is common in young people, and 75% of perforating injuries occur in patients under the age of 30; a third of these will be children under the age of 10 years. In the adult group there is a male preponderance of 3:1.

In the last 25 years the proportion of injuries occurring in the home or from child play has remained relatively constant, while occupational injuries have fallen because of improved safety precautions. Windscreen injuries showed a huge increase between 1959 and 1981; the introduction of seat-belt legislation has significantly reduced this problem. Assault is now the most common cause of penetrating eye injuries.

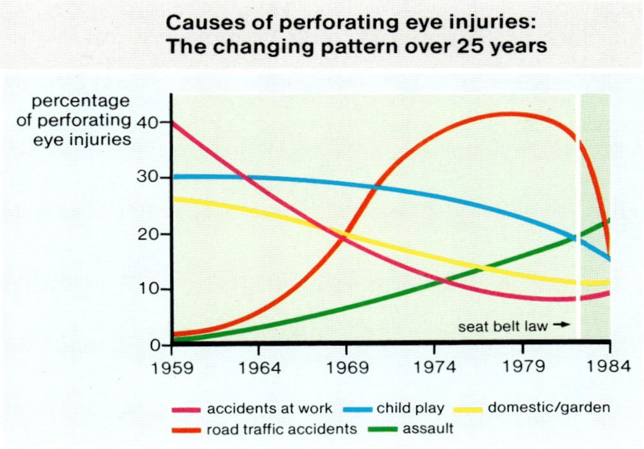

**Causes of perforating eye injuries:
The changing pattern over 25 years**

percentage of perforating eye injuries

seat belt law →

1959 1964 1969 1974 1979 1984

■ accidents at work ■ child play ■ domestic/garden
■ road traffic accidents ■ assault

Fig.6.4 The changing pattern of injury over 25 years.

Recognition of Perforating Eye Injuries

A perforation of the eye should always be suspected when an accident involving a sharp object has occurred. Often the injury is localised to the eye, but in some situations other injuries may be present that require immediate treatment; the patient should be placed in a recumbent position and a general assessment of all injuries must be made before a detailed ocular examination is carried out. Treatment of any life-threatening complication has priority.

History

The *history* of the injury is of great importance: a detailed description of the accident should be recorded, noting the time of the accident, how it was caused and what action was taken immediately afterwards. If available, the instrument that caused the injury should be examined, as this may provide clues regarding the depth of penetration. Injuries involving organic material, such as thorns, carry a higher risk of infection, while those from broken glass may have left particles within the eye. If the causative agent is still present, care must be taken not to aggravate the injury before repair can be undertaken.

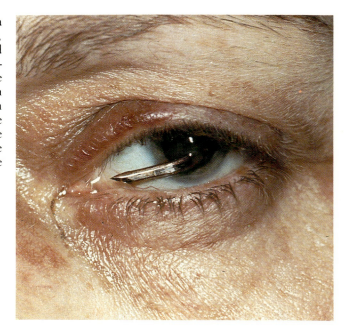

Fig.6.5 Piece of staple causing a perforating injury. By courtesy of Mr. J.B. Garston.

Examination

Assessment of vision is important, as outlined in Chapter 1 (see page 1.3); in severe injuries the absence of light perception or defective light projection carries a grave prognosis.

Preliminary examination with focal illumination is carried out (see pages 1.4–5). The injury may be obvious; an extensive laceration, hyphaema and obvious prolapse of tissues (see Fig.6.1) should be disturbed as little as possible prior to repair. The injury should be covered with a light dressing and the patient given an anti-emetic and analgesic injection to prevent further damage from vomiting and restlessness.

x

Slit-lamp examination

In the less extensive injuries, particularly those confined to the anterior segment, examination on the slit-lamp provides much additional information. The extent and nature of the wound can be confirmed and damage to underlying tissues may be visible, if not obscured by internal bleeding.

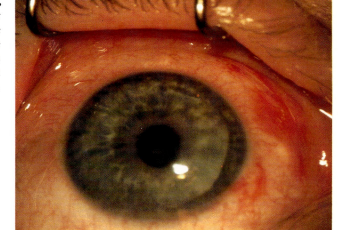

The simplest wound is a linear laceration of the cornea, with loss of the anterior chamber. If the anterior chamber is flat, this is obvious to naked eye examination, but if the anterior chamber has partly reformed, the depth of the wound can be assessed on the slit-lamp and aqueous leakage can be confirmed by applying a sterile fluorescein paper to the wound and observing streaming of the dye.

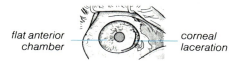

Fig.6.6 Simple corneal laceration with flat anterior chamber.

Puncture from an object like a crochet hook or pencil causes a stellate wound of the cornea; if the centre of the cornea is affected, iris prolapse is unlikely but lens damage is common. A layer of fibrin across the pupil may mimic this, and a further examination should always be made after dilating the pupil with 1% cyclopentolate. Breaks in the lens capsule can then be confirmed while fibrin separates from the pupil and is identified in front of the lens.

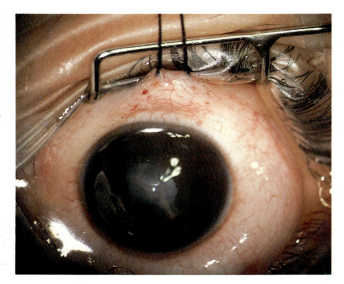

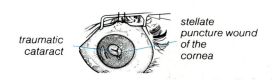

Fig.6.7 Stellate puncture wound of the cornea with traumatic cataract.

Puncture wounds or lacerations near the limbus are commonly associated with iris prolapse; this results in a pear-shaped pupil and a knuckle of iris may be visible in the wound. In such an injury the iris tissue may be strangulated in the wound, becoming oedematous and rigid. This makes surgical repositioning difficult.

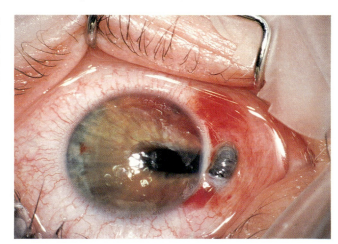

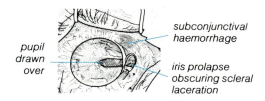

Fig.6.8 Oedematous iris prolapse in a limbal wound.

A small puncture wound of the cornea from an object like a thorn may become sealed and the anterior chamber reformed; the patient may be unaware of the extent of the injury until progressive cataract formation leads to diminished vision, or inflammation develops.

Larger lacerations of the cornea may have a complex pattern with extension into the sclera on one or both sides of the limbus. The laceration is often shelving with stellate or Y-shaped branches. The anterior chamber is lost, and with persisting hypotony the wound becomes progressively oedematous, making accurate suturing difficult. Both iris and lens damage may be present and the extent of the injury may be obscured by bleeding within the eye (see also Fig.6.1).

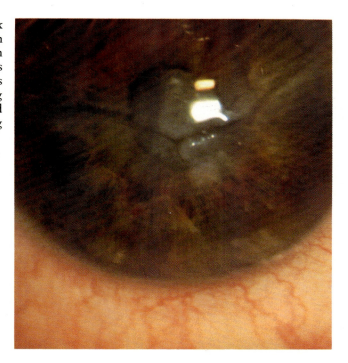

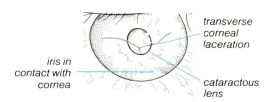

Fig.6.9 Branching laceration of the cornea with traumatic cataract.

Clean lacerations confined to the sclera are relatively uncommon; in the absence of haemorrhage, prolapsed vitreous gel with surrounding uveal pigment may be visible through a posterior wound (see Fig.6.21).

Most scleral wounds are an extension of a corneal laceration or a limbal rupture, and usually involve the ciliary body region. The dark uveal prolapse is often visible, but haemorrhage under the conjunctiva makes identification of damaged tissues difficult. The full extent of a scleral laceration is often obscured, and will only be revealed by exposure during repair.

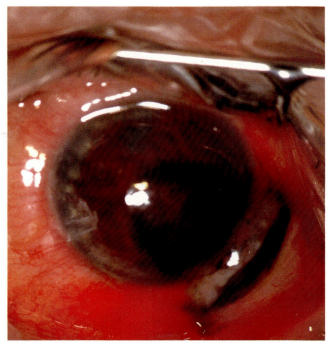

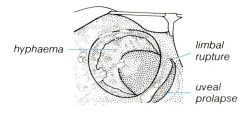

Fig.6.10 Laceration of the sclera with uveal prolapse and hyphaema.

Very extensive lacerations and ruptures leave a collapsed globe with expulsion of iris, lens and vitreous; major haemorrhage from the choroidal vessels may also occur with prolapse of retina into the wound (see Fig.6.25, page 6.12). Continued bleeding often makes identification of tissues very difficult.

Planning the Surgical Repair

As repair will involve general anaesthesia, some delay will usually result until the patient is fit for surgery. During this period it is important to keep the patient as still as possible, protecting the injured eye with a light dressing. The patient will be in a state of anxiety and shock, and may need sedation and anti-emetic treatment. The extent of the injury and the prognosis should be explained; our policy is always to attempt primary repair, so although the visual prognosis may be guarded, any question of removing the eye should be deferred to a later date.

An x-ray examination is desirable as this may reveal retained fragments of glass or other material within the globe. In a severe injury, a portable x-ray should be requested to avoid moving the patient. Tetanus prophylaxis should be given as outlined in Chapter 1 (see page 1.3) as well as parenteral antibiotics.

The aims of surgery are to *remove* disorganised tissue and debris, *reposit* viable tissue such as iris or retina, *repair* the wound to give a watertight closure, and *restore* anatomical relationships of the anterior and posterior segments. The approach will differ depending on the site and extent of the wound, and the presence of internal bleeding. It is convenient to discuss the repair of injuries in three categories: those confined to the anterior segment (with iris and lens damage, but no vitreous loss), those confined to the posterior segment (with vitreous loss but no lens damage), and the extensive injuries involving both anterior and posterior segments.

Principles of repair

1. REMOVE disorganised tissue and haemorrhage.

2. REPOSIT viable tissue such as iris.

3. REPAIR the wound accurately.

4. RESTORE anatomical relationships.

Some general considerations

In any penetrating injury the extent of damage should be reassessed once the patient is anaesthetised. Where both eye and facial lacerations are present, the eye injury should be repaired first. The eyelashes should not be cut when an open wound of the globe is present; they may be covered by using a sterile adhesive drape. In children it is safest to use lid sutures for retraction of the eyelids or individual retractors strapped in position; this avoids exerting any pressure on the globe which might occur with the introduction of a speculum.

Adequate exposure of the wound is an essential part of repair. In a collapsed eye it is unsafe to introduce tract-ion sutures under the rectus muscles, as the globe may be perforated by the needle. Two or more limbal sutures are placed, using 0.7 metric (6/0) silk.

At the completion of repair a subconjunctival injection of methicillin 150 mg is given; in contaminated wounds gentamicin 40 mg is given as well. In injuries with lens damage, a subconjunctival injection of betamethasone 4 mg is also given. Antibiotic and 1% atropine drops are instilled, and the eye is covered with a tulle gras dressing, plus an eye pad and shield. Postoperative analgesic and anti-emetic treatment is prescribed, and systemic antibiotics are continued.

Repair of Anterior Segment Perforations

Some of these injuries will have a wound which has sealed spontaneously or is plugged by iris prolapse. If the anterior chamber is present, it is helpful to make an initial *paracentesis* in the cornea near to the wound using a very sharp blade (see Fig.6.13). The paracentesis is required later for reforming the anterior chamber. It is easier to do this before disturbing the wound and losing intraocular pressure; if however the wound is wide open, this step is deferred until later in the repair.

Some injuries may have a dangerous spicule of glass or other agent protruding into the anterior chamber, with a risk of further damage to internal structures during repair. A paracentesis will allow deepening of the anterior chamber at an early stage using sodium hyaluronate; this visco-elastic substance is retained in the anterior chamber during repair giving extra protection to vital structures.

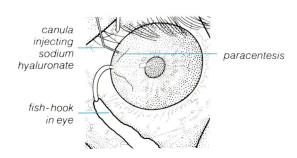

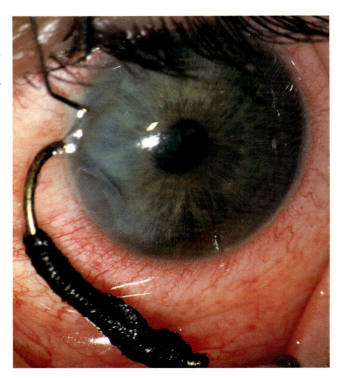

Fig.6.11 Fish-hook penetrating the anterior chamber; depth is increased with sodium hyaluronate via a paracentesis.

Wound exposure and management of iris prolapse

The first step is to identify the extent and nature of the wound; if this is confined to the cornea, the extent is clearly visible under the operating microscope. The wound may be shelving in depth and direction; gentle inspection using either a fine irrigating canula and balanced salt solution or lifting with tissue forceps will help identify the outline of the wound.

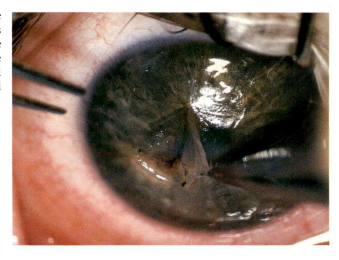

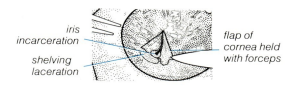

Fig.6.12 Shelving corneal laceration with iris incarceration.

Any contamination should be cleaned from the wound by irrigation and the viability of an iris prolapse is tested with compressed cellulose sponges; if it disintegrates, it is non-viable and should be abscised. The disorganised tissue is lifted with a cellulose sponge or fine toothed forceps and cut away using iris scissors.

Healthy iris tissue should be returned to the anterior chamber; the iris prolapse is freed via a paracentesis, deepening the anterior chamber with sodium hyaluronate and sweeping the synechia with an angled repositor or the tip of a fine canula.

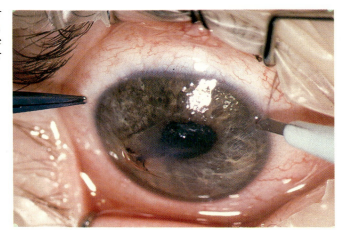

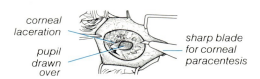

Fig.6.13 Paracentesis prepared for releasing iris incarceration.

Wound repair (see page 6.8) is then carried out and any residual iris adhesion is freed from the wound. Sodium hyaluronate can be aspirated or diluted with balanced salt solution; air should be removed at the end of the procedure and the anterior chamber reformed with balanced salt solution. The wound is then checked with a compressed cellulose sponge to confirm a watertight closure.

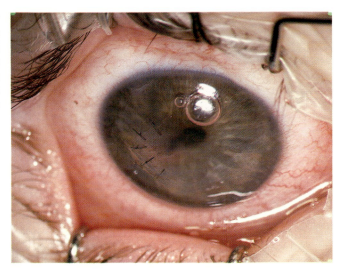

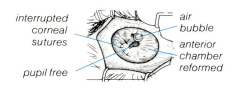

Fig.6.14 Wound repair completed in the above injury.

An iris prolapse into a small limbal wound (Fig.6.8) will be difficult to reposit; it may be necessary to enlarge the wound in order to return the prolapse to the anterior chamber. An angled repositor is used via a paracentesis (Fig.6.13) and a solution of 1% acetylcholine is injected into the anterior chamber to constrict the pupil. Because of atonicity, the peripheral portion of the iris should be abscised to avoid wound synechiae.

Lacerations extending from the cornea into the anterior sclera are often complicated by iris prolapse along the length of the wound; a layer of fibrin covering the prolapse makes it adherent to the wound. The tissue should be freed by injecting sodium hyaluronate or by gently passing a repositor between the wound and the prolapse on either side: any devitalised iris tissue should be abscised. To expose the scleral wound, the conjunc-tiva is grasped at the limbus on either side and cut with fine spring-action scissors for a short distance around the limbus. The apex of the conjunctival wound is extended and Tenon's capsule is freed from the wound by spreading the scissors gently between the sclera and overlying tissues. Superficial bleeding is common during exposure and should be controlled by wet-field bipolar cautery.

If healthy, the central portion of an iris prolapse should be returned to the anterior chamber and held back with a repositor during suturing. The peripheral iris should always be abscised through the wound, otherwise an anterior synechia will occur at this point.

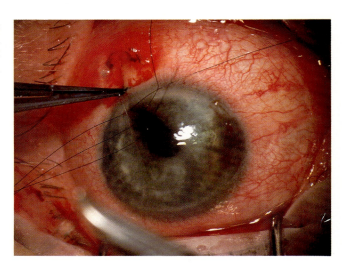

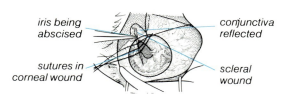

Fig.6.15 Wound exposure in a limbal perforation; damaged iris abscised.

Wound repair is then carried out (see below) and the anterior chamber is reformed via a separate paracentesis, otherwise iris tissue may be forced back into the wound. If synechiae to the wound persist, air or sodium hyaluronate are used to help separate the tissues, or an angled repositor may be required. The anterior chamber is then reformed with balanced salt solution.

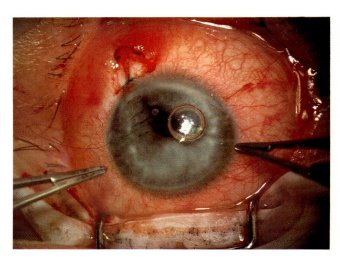

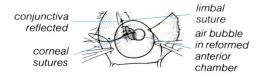

Fig.6.16 Wound repair completed and anterior chamber restored.

Where possible, an iris prolapse should be reposited rather than abscised, otherwise a large sector iridectomy will result in an unsightly appearance and cause photophobia and monocular diplopia. This particularly occurs if the defect is in the lower temporal quadrant.

The main risk of repositing an iris prolapse is intro-ducing infection (there is no evidence that repositing an iris prolapse increases the risk of sympathetic ophthalmitis). The risk of introducing infection increases with time, and if repair is undertaken more than 24 hours after injury, any prolapsed tissue should be completely excised even if viable. Prolapsed iris should always be abscised if the wound is dirty or infection is already present.

Wound repair

A simple linear laceration of the cornea can be closed by interrupted 0.2 metric (10/0) nylon sutures; when the wound crosses the limbus, this should be aligned immediately after cleaning and identifying any scleral extension. The accuracy of this stitch is very important, otherwise disastrous astigmatism may result from malalignment.

Corneal sutures are then placed at intervals across the wound; once two or three sutures have been placed, the anterior chamber should be deepened with sodium hyal-uronate, as restoring the shape of the eye will help to align the tissues accurately. The sutures should be of the correct width and depth, and ultimately spaced not more than 2 mm apart. After wound closure the knots are buried by rotating them in the suture track to avoid irritation (see Fig.6.16), and the watertightness of the wound is confirmed by testing it with a compressed cellulose sponge.

An oedematous or shelving wound is difficult to suture accurately; in the former, a common mistake is to place the sutures either too wide or too shallow, resulting in flattening of the wound and poor apposition of the deeper layers. In a shelving wound (see Fig.6.12), the stitch should be a longer bite for the overhanging flap, otherwise the deeper aspect will not be closed.

Stellate wounds (see Fig.6.7) are often difficult to seal: in this situation a purse string or mattress suture is needed. If close to the axis of vision, with no prolapse and minimal leakage, it is preferable to bandage with a soft contact lens as suturing such a wound may leave a prominent scar.

Fine monofilament nylon sutures should be left in situ for at least six months, unless they become loose and are protruding.

Fig.6.17 Diagrams showing the correct placement of sutures for linear and stellate lacerations, and the effect of incorrectly placed sutures.

Management of lens damage

Unless capsule rupture has been clearly identified, lens surgery during primary repair should not be attempted. Where it is clear that the lens capsule has been disrupted, it is preferable to complete lens surgery during the primary repair, otherwise rapid swelling of the lens may cause synechia to the wound in the postoperative period and subsequent surgery may be associated with excessive endothelial damage.

Flocculent lens matter can be washed away during the repair of the wound, but in most cases definitive lens surgery is performed after completing the wound closure. The pupil is dilated by topical 1.0% cyclopentolate instilled at the commencement of repair.

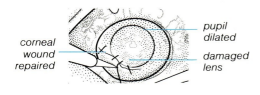

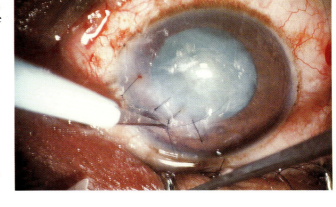

Fig.6.18 Primary repair of corneal laceration completed; the pupil has been dilated at the commencement of surgery.

The age of the patient will determine whether lens aspiration or an extracapsular lens extraction is required. Pupil dilation is assisted by irrigating the anterior chamber with 1/100,000 adrenaline (diluting intracardiac adrenaline in 500 ml of balanced salt solution). It is helpful to use a cutting device, as removal of capsule remnants is often required. The techniques are discussed further in Chapter 8 (see pages 8.5–7).

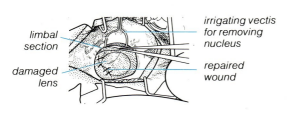

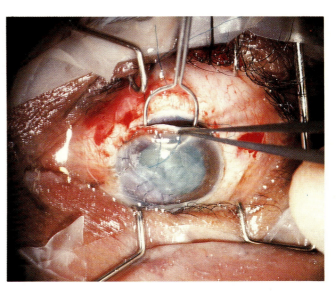

Fig.6.19 Extracapsular extraction in the above injury.

Postoperative management

The result of primary surgery should be assessed in the immediate postoperative period. Infection is extremely rare, but may develop within 48 hours, requiring vigorous treatment (see also page 7.10). If anterior synechiae to the wound remain secondary surgery is advisable, otherwise this will cause intense fibrovascular invasion of the wound and lead to a dense scar with severe astigmatism. Lens rupture may not have been evident at the time of repair but if present it will lead to rapid cataract formation; secondary surgical inter-vention should be prompt.

In children it is very important to achieve clear media and optical correction as soon as possible after the injury; primary lens surgery will allow optical correction within a very short period. In young children, padding of the injured eye should be discontinued at the first dressing. Both astigmatism and aphakia will cause rapid amblyopia, and the refraction should be checked as soon as possible. Astigmatism should be corrected with glasses in the first instance.

After cataract removal, the vision can be corrected with a continuous wear soft contact lens within a few days of surgery. In children, the vision in the injured eye will need to be maintained with occlusion treatment, and continuing orthoptic supervision is very important.

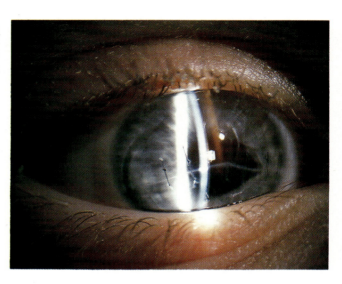

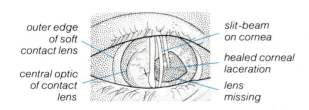

Fig.6.20 Contact lens fitted two weeks after traumatic aphakia.

Perforating Injuries Confined to the Posterior Segment

These are relatively uncommon injuries consisting of scleral lacerations with damage confined to the posterior segment. (Although ruptures of the globe commonly affect the sclera only, these are almost always associated with an expulsive injury and anterior segment damage as well). Small scleral wounds, particularly those situated in the pars plana, will have vitreous prolapse but little or no internal haemorrhage; larger lacerations that extend posteriorly to involve choroid and retina have a higher incidence of vitreous haemorrhage, which leads to complications.

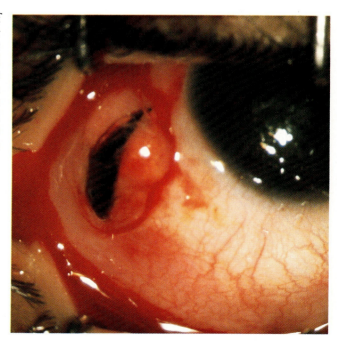

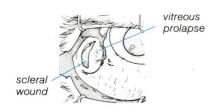

Fig.6.21 Scleral laceration with vitreous prolapse.

Surgical management

Before commencing the repair, 1% cyclopentolate drops should be instilled to dilate the pupil, so that fundus examination can be performed at the end of the repair.

The wound is exposed as described earlier (see page 6.8); an accurate description of the position and posterior extent of the wound should be recorded, using calipers to measure the distance behind the limbus. Wounds extending more than 6 mm posteriorly will involve the vitreous base and retina.

After exposing the wound, prolapsed vitreous gel is abscised. In posterior wounds this should be performed very gently, using compressed cellulose sponges to lift the gel and abscising flush with the wound.

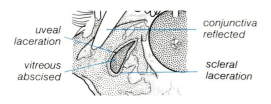

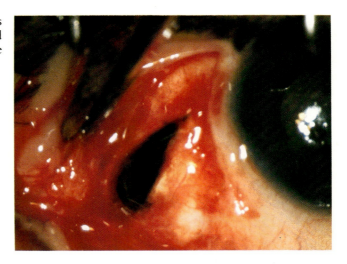

Fig.6.22 Scleral wound exposed and vitreous prolapse abscised.

When abscising prolapsed vitreous, it is important not to introduce a sponge too deeply into the wound, as the gel will still be adherent to retina, and traction on this may pull retina or pars plana into the wound. If available, a vitreous cutter can clean the wound more safely. Once clean, the wound is then closed using interrupted 0.3 metric (9/0) nylon or 0.4 metric (8/0) virgin silk sutures. Further abscision of vitreous strands may be required during wound closure. Finally the conjunctiva is repaired using 0.7 metric (6/0) collagen.

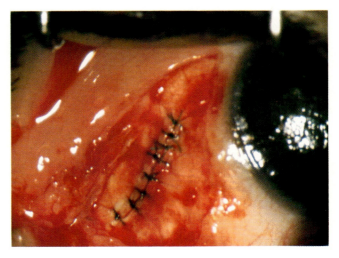

Fig.6.23 Closure of the scleral wound with interrupted silk sutures.

The volume of the globe may need restoring, and as in anterior segment injuries this is best performed at a site remote from the wound. In a soft eye good fixation is required, using the insertion of one of the rectus muscles on the side opposite to the wound. A small conjunctival incision is made 4 mm behind the limbus, and a fine-gauged needle is introduced into the centre of the vitreous cavity using counter traction on the muscle insertion; balanced salt solution rather than air is used to restore intraocular pressure, so that visibility of the posterior segment can be maintained. Sodium hyaluronate may prove to be useful in this context as an alternative replacement fluid.

Examination of the posterior segment should now be carried out with the indirect ophthalmoscope. Vitreous haemorrhage may obscure the view; the extent of this should be recorded, as it is an important parameter in the subsequent management. In the absence of haemorrhage, the relationship of the vitreous base near the wound can be seen. If gel incarceration is still present, the adjacent vitreous base is elevated, lifting both retina and choroid. If left like this, small oral breaks will subsequently occur and allow retinal detachment. If this appearance is seen, the wound will require revision.

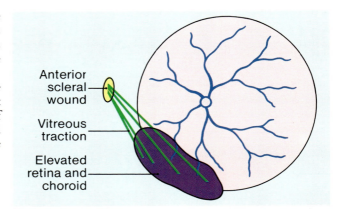

Fig.6.24 Diagram illustrating gel incarceration and traction.

Cryotherapy of the wound is not advocated, as this may precipitate haemorrhage. Even if the wound extends into the retina, chorioretinal scarring at this point provides strong adhesion, and the retinal wound does not directly cause retinal detachment (this is usually the result of traction from gel incarceration). Cryotherapy is, however, recommended two to four weeks after injury to the adjacent vitreous base, to protect against oral breaks.

Management of retinal prolapse

One problem that may occasionally occur is a full-thickness scleral wound that has *not cut through* the underlying uveoretinal tissue. A rise of intraocular pressure causes prolapse of intact retina into the wound but the absence of major haemorrhage is indicated by the normal translucent appearance of the prolapsed tissues. If vitrectomy facilities are available, it may be possible to reposit the prolapsed retina after a pars plana vitrectomy (see Chapters 7 and 9). If not available, an anterior chamber paracentesis should be performed to reduce intraocular pressure, but any residual retinal prolapse must be abscised to try and prevent incarceration. The vitreous cavity is then distended with air to help restore the normal anatomical relationships, and sodium hyaluronate is introduced via the wound. Some incarceration often remains, and prognosis for retaining vision is poor as epiretinal fibrosis and retinal detachment are likely.

Retinal prolapse is more often present if a major suprachoroidal haemorrhage has occurred. Blood is evident on either side of the prolapse, which appears dark from additional bleeding within the cavity. Attempted repositioning is a hopeless task, and the prolapse has to be abscised. The eye usually becomes phthisical.

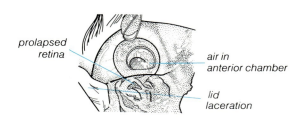

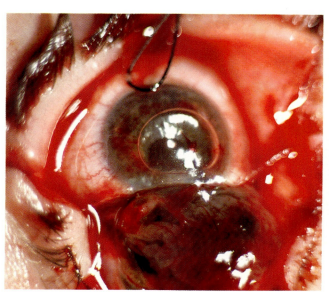

Fig.6.25 Haemorrhagic retinal prolapse through a scleral laceration. By courtesy of Miss E.E. Kritzinger.

Postoperative management of scleral lacerations

Bed rest should be maintained for four days in injuries accompanied by vitreous haemorrhage; recurrent vitreous and suprachoroidal haemorrhage is common in the early postoperative period. Early assessment of the posterior segment is important to check that no gel incarceration remains (see Fig.6.24). The appearance is similar to a choroidal detachment but with obvious gel traction to the wound. If present, early vitrectomy under indirect control is required, otherwise traction detachment will follow (see page 9.4).

Peripheral gel haemorrhage is the commonest complication and leads to localised tangential traction developing in the vitreous base. This takes place slowly over several months, and can be monitored by examination with the indirect ophthalmoscope.

Prophylactic cryotherapy (page 6.11) helps prevent detachment, but if the peripheral retina shows signs of lifting, an encircling procedure will be required; the wound should also be indented by a radial sponge. The changes are slow to develop, and retinal detachment surgery is rarely required before three months have elapsed.

Diffuse vitreous haemorrhage is most often seen with a wound extending posteriorly into the retina. It is a potent stimulus to fibroplasia, which extends along the posterior surface of the detached vitreous cortex and locally on the surface of the retina. Fibroblasts invade from the wound, as it is impossible to avoid some gel incarceration at this point. Ultimately, contraction of membranes leads to traction detachment.

If the view of the retina is totally obscured in the postoperative period, vitrectomy is indicated to prevent traction detachment. Since diffuse vitreous haemorrhage indicates some degree of contusion, surgery is planned between four and six weeks after injury. This subject is discussed in more detail in Chapter 9 (see page 9.4).

Compound Injuries involving both Anterior and Posterior Segments

Management of injuries without major internal haemorrhage

These injuries represent the more anterior lacerations involving cornea and sclera, with iris damage and rupture of the lens accompanied by vitreous prolapse. Hyphaema may be present but is not filling the anterior chamber, and active bleeding from the scleral part of the wound is not present. At one end of the spectrum, the lens diaphragm has only partly been disrupted and, although vitreous prolapse is present, the globe is not collapsed. In these injuries it is important to deal adequately with the lens-vitreous mixture, otherwise a cyclitic membrane will form, leading to hypotony and eventual retinal detachment.

6.12

In the more extensive injuries, the lens has often been expelled and the globe has collapsed. The retina may be prolapsing towards the wound, and is sometimes visible in the anterior chamber. This can occur in young patients with an extensive laceration because of the lack of rigidity of the tissues. Internal prolapse of the retina may occur without major internal haemorrhage or retinal disruption, and anatomical replacement with normal retinal function can be achieved.

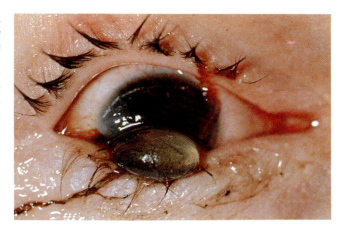

Fig.6.26 Extensive laceration with prolapse of intraocular contents: the intact lens is lying on the surface. By courtesy of Mr. J.B. Garston.

Surgical management

The extent of the wound is identified as described earlier, and a preliminary assessment of the internal damage is made. When the wound extends into the sclera, a single 0.3 metric (9/0) nylon suture is placed to *align the limbus*, taking care to avoid any incarceration of tissues by holding these back with a repositor. Any damaged tissues prolapsing through the corneal wound are then excised; gentle irrigation of the anterior chamber is carried out to clear away any hyphaema and flocculent lens matter.

The presence of vitreous prolapse can be confirmed by its characteristic adhesion to compressed cellulose sponges: this should be excised with caution, as in a collapsed eye; retina may be prolapsing towards the anterior chamber and can be pulled into the wound.

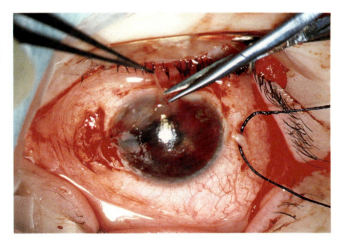

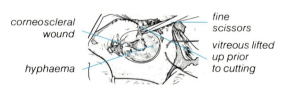

corneoscleral wound

hyphaema

fine scissors

vitreous lifted up prior to cutting

Fig.6.27 Corneoscleral laceration; vitreous prolapse being abscised.

A manual technique for removing prolapsing vitreous using compressed cellulose sponges is often effective, but it is difficult to deal with a disrupted lens, as the presence of vitreous makes aspiration impossible. Where large amounts of lens matter mixed with vitreous remain, the use of a vitreous cutter will facilitate removal. This is best performed after wound closure using a bimanual technique via two small limbal incisions (see page 7.8).

As soon as the corneal wound is clean, a few interrupted full-thickness sutures are placed in the cornea using 0.2 metric (10/0) nylon. Air is then introduced into the anterior chamber to restore the shape of the globe; this is supplemented with sodium hyaluronate which helps retain the air. Repair of the corneal wound is then completed after checking that no further prolapse of tissue is present; the knots should be buried by rotating them into the suture track.

The reason for repairing the corneal would first, followed by air tamponade, is to avoid incarcerating tissue in the scleral part of the wound. Having restored the shape of the globe and hopefully having replaced any prolapsed pars plana and retina, the scleral part of the wound can be repaired using 0.3 metric (9/0) nylon; the knots should be cut short to avoid irritation. Apart from tags of iris, tissues in this part of the wound should not be abscised but held back with a repositor while suturing the laceration.

Fig.6.28 Air tamponade of the globe prior to repairing sclera.

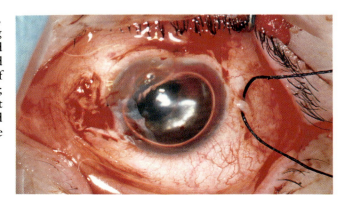

After completing the wound repair, the air should be replaced with a balanced salt solution, so that the water-tightness of the wound can be confirmed. The anterior chamber is inspected, and if any lens matter is still remaining, lensectomy plus anterior vitrectomy can now be performed (see pages 8.6-7 for details of this technique).

The importance of dealing adequately with a damaged lens mixed with blood and vitreous cannot be over-emphasised. Failure to remove these tissues encourages fibrosis with a cyclitic membrane that causes ciliary body detachment and hypotony, and eventually leads to retinal detachment and phthisis bulbi.

In those patients where lens and vitreous have been expulsed and internal prolapse of retina has been identified, the air should be left in situ to provide tamponade to the retina over several days.

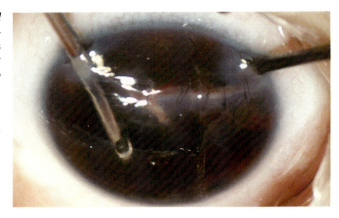

Fig.6.29 Lensectomy at the completion of repair.

Postoperatively there may be complications of either the anterior or posterior segments: residual lens matter may need further surgery if a significant amount remains. Lensectomy is the treatment of choice as this technique can deal with capsule remnants and any synechiae to the wound, plus removing the anterior vitreous. The posterior segment needs careful assessment when the view is sufficiently clear, as some of these injuries may have vitreous haemorrhage or peripheral retinal pathology. These techniques are described in more detail in Chapters 8 and 9.

Management of injuries with major internal haemorrhage

This category of injury carries the worst prognosis, and includes almost all eyes which have suffered severe contusion leading to a ruptured globe. Expulsion of intraocular contents occurs with haemorrhage into the subretinal and suprachoroidal spaces. The eye is full of blood and often the retina has prolapsed. There is usually no light perception present prior to repair.

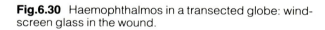

Fig.6.30 Haemophthalmos in a transected globe: windscreen glass in the wound.

Although it is usually clear from the extent of damage that restoration of sight or even a reasonable cosmetic appearance is unlikely, our policy is to attempt repair, as the outcome is occasionally better than expected; this policy also allows time for the patient to adjust to the situation before enucleation for a blind and unsightly eye is recommended.

Not all these eyes are damaged beyond recovery, and those with a more anterior wound without external prolapse of retina can regain good function even though they appear full of blood initially. The management is similar to that described earlier (page 6.13); because of expulsion of intraocular contents, there is usually no remaining lens or vitreous but bleeding often continues from within the eye. The aim should be to place a few controlling sutures as soon as possible, so that air tamponade can restore intraocular pressure and help control further haemorrhage. In these extensive injuries the air should be left in situ, to provide tamponade to the posterior segment over several days.

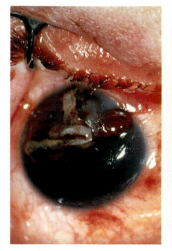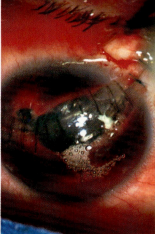

Fig.6.31 left Corneoscleral laceration with internal haemorrhage.
Fig.6.31 right Air tamponade after repair.

In these injuries, after repairing the laceration and restoring intraocular pressure with air, a suprachoroidal tap should be made on either side of the wound in the pars plana region. An incision is made through the sclera to expose the underlying uvea, and gentle irrigation via the wound is carried out. The aim is to provide potential drainage for suprachoroidal haemorrhage: the blood has usually clotted by this time, so it cannot be washed out, but the incisions should be left unsutured to allow escape of altered blood when it subsequently liquefies. Air tamponade should be repeated after this procedure.

Many of these eyes end up blind and are removed; subsequent histology confirms extensive suprachoroidal and subretinal haemorrhage. The latter leads to rapid disorganisation and fibrosis and is not amenable to surgical treatment.

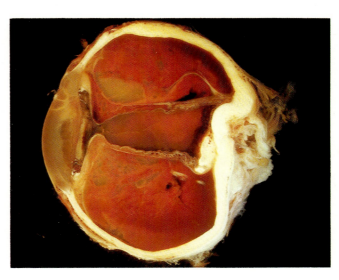

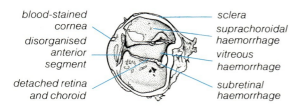

Fig.6.32 Suprachoroidal and subretinal haemorrhage in an eye enucleated ten days after a perforating injury. By courtesy of Prof. W.R. Lee.

Postoperative management

As these eyes have suffered a contusion injury, bed rest should be continued in the postoperative period for several days. Sudden pain and a rise of intraocular pressure suggests further bleeding within the eye. In many of these eyes the anterior chamber remains filled with blood for days, but by the end of one week some red reflex may be visible on slit-lamp examination.

Posterior segment haemorrhage is common, and will take several weeks to clear. These eyes often have little or no remaining iris, and the lens and vitreous have usually been expelled.

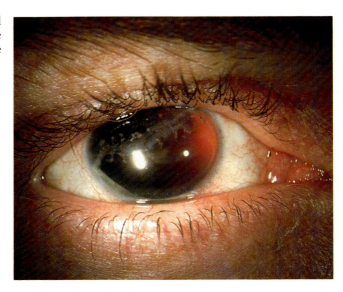

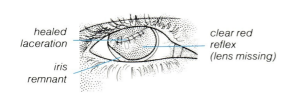

Fig.6.33 Aniridia and aphakia after a perforating injury (see Fig.6.31 for appearance at time of repair).

In the postoperative period, a careful watch should be kept on the level of vision; in these severe injuries it is often reduced to doubtful light perception, but even this may improve as suprachoroidal and subretinal haemorrhage absorbs. Usually a downward trend to no light perception occurs, with the eye rapidly becoming irritable and shrunken; ultrasonography will help confirm the disorganisation of tissues within the eye, while electrodiagnostic tests give additional information on retinal function (see page 7.2). Enucleation is advisable where there is no hope of visual recovery, so that rehabilitation may be quickly achieved and the very small risk of sympathetic ophthalmitis avoided.

In those eyes that retain accurate light projection and normal pressure, a conservative approach is adopted; vitrectomy for diffuse vitreous haemorrhage may need to be considered to prevent traction retinal detachment, but because a major contusion element has been present, this is usually deferred for four to six weeks. In practice, since vitreous has usually been totally expelled, vitrectomy is rarely required, but peripheral retinal damage and local incarceration in the wound may need retinal surgery (see page 9.4).

With injuries *confined to the anterior segment* the prognosis for retaining the injured eye and achieving good vision is excellent. Infection occasionally leads to loss of an eye, particularly if presentation has been delayed or the wound is contaminated by organic material. The complications of wound fistulae, incarceration of tissues anteriorly and epithelial ingrowth have become rare and should be avoided (for management see page 8.15).

Eyes without lens damage should recover normal vision; wound scarring and astigmatism may detract from the final visual outcome in some patients, particularly in the larger wounds that cross the limbus. Factors contributing to this may be poor surgical technique (incorrect suturing or anterior synechiae to the wound), or failure in the postoperative period to remove loose or irritating sutures; all these factors stimulate vascular invasion of the wound, leading to fibrosis and flattening of the cornea and resulting in high astigmatism.

Injuries *with lens damage to one eye only* can have a technically satisfactory outcome, but maintenance of comfortable binocular vision with contact lens wear is rare, particularly in the younger age group. Despite primary lens surgery and early fitting of contact lenses, few patients continue to wear them after the first year. Children under the age of six rapidly become amblyopic despite orthoptic treatment, while even the older age group diverge very quickly.

If secondary lens surgery is undertaken in the early period after injury, an intraocular lens implant can be inserted; this should only be performed when the posterior capsule is intact and vitreous has not been lost; a posterior chamber implant is the lens of choice. Children may react badly to this procedure as postoperative inflammation is common and fibroplasia may be severe. In the young age group a safe but amblyopic eye may have to be accepted.

Those already aphakic will usually undergo a trial of contact lens wear (see Fig.6.20); if this proves unacceptable, a secondary implantation of an intraocular lens may be considered. An anterior chamber lens is the most suitable in this situation. The management of traumatic aphakia and other anterior segment reconstruction is considered in detail later (see page 8.5).

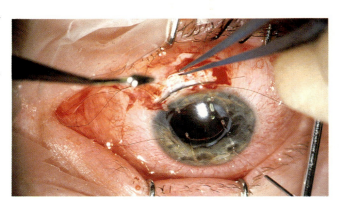

Fig.6.34 Inserting a secondary anterior chamber implant for traumatic aphakia.

Injuries involving anterior and posterior segments have a poor outcome, reflecting the high incidence of expulsive haemorrhage. In our last review, 60% of these eyes became blind or were excised. Retention of vision depends on the absence of major internal bleeding and spontaneous expulsion of the lens or radical anterior segment surgery. The contusion element causes angle damage; retinal problems and late glaucoma may be encountered.

In *injuries confined to the posterior segment*, the visual outcome is good in the absence of major haemorrhage. Vitreous haemorrhage stimulates intraocular fibrosis and leads to traction retinal detachment. In some cases, this may be localised to the periphery and controlled by cryotherapy or encircling procedures, but those associated with diffuse vitreous haemorrhage will develop extensive traction. Vitreous surgery helps to prevent this complication (see page 9.3).

In extensive injuries, aphakia combined with aniridia leaves an eye that is very photophobic; both an improved cosmetic appearance and optical correction can be achieved with painted haptic lenses.

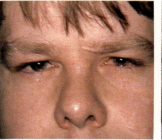 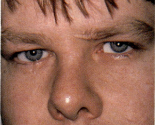

Fig.6.35 left Bilateral perforating injuries with aphakia and aniridia.
Fig.6.35 right Same patient with painted haptic contact lenses.

Many of these injured eyes come to enucleation, not because of the risk of sympathetic ophthalmitis, but because they are disorganised and likely to remain irritable and unsightly. Sympathetic ophthalmitis is now an extremely rare complication of penetrating eye injuries (in our last review it occurred in less than 0.5% of injuries), but where there is no prospect of recovering any vision, that risk should not be ignored, and the injured eye should be enucleated within two weeks of injury. (For further discussion see page 7.11).

INTRAOCULAR FOREIGN BODIES

Recognition of these injuries is very important, as failure to detect and remove a foreign body within the first 24 hours may result in complications that lead to blindness in the affected eye.

Causes of Injury

The majority of injuries result from hammering steel on steel, but some result from hammering bricks or concrete. The particle that penetrates the eye has usually come off the hammer or chisel and, if available, both tools should be inspected. As these are steel particles, they are magnetic. Machine tool accidents also result in steel fragments penetrating the eye; injuries from explosions lead to ragged particles (usually non-magnetic) penetrating the eye. Air-gun pellets can also occasionally penetrate the eye.

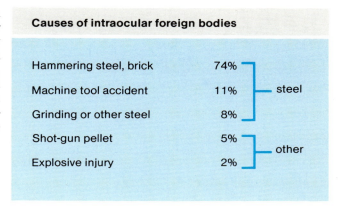

Causes of intraocular foreign bodies

Hammering steel, brick	74%	steel
Machine tool accident	11%	
Grinding or other steel	8%	
Shot-gun pellet	5%	other
Explosive injury	2%	

Fig.6.36 Table showing causes of intraocular foreign bodies in a recent review at our hospital.

Presentation

The history is vital in recognising these injuries; any patient who presents with a history of something hitting the eye while using a hammer should be presumed to have an intraocular foreign body until proved otherwise.

With *large foreign bodies* an open eye injury occurs, usually accompanied by considerable internal bleeding. The severity of injury is obvious (see Fig.6.3).

With *small foreign bodies* the symptoms may be minimal: the entry wound is often small and seals spontaneously, so there may be little or no visual disturbance and no discomfort in the early stages. The commonest symptom is 'floaters' from a disturbance of the vitreous by a posterior segment foreign body.

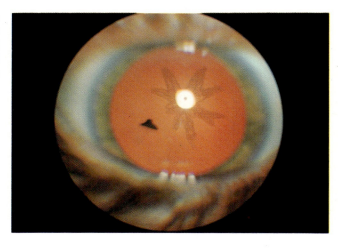

Fig.6.37 Vitreous haemorrhage in a posterior segment foreign body.

If the injury is not recognised, the patient may present a day or two later because of progressive lens changes leading to reduced vision. The particle has usually passed right through the lens, but occasionally it is arrested within the lens substance. A posterior rosette cataract is often the first sign of progressive opacification.

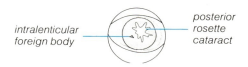

intralenticular foreign body — posterior rosette cataract

Fig.6.38 Rosette cataract with an intralenticular foreign body.

In some cases a painful red eye develops after one or two days due to an acute exudative uveitis; marked photophobia and lacrimation are present. Vision is profoundly reduced and a hypopyon may be present in the anterior chamber.

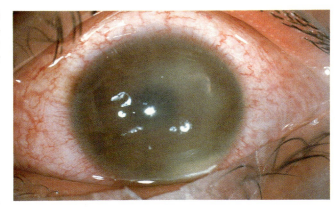

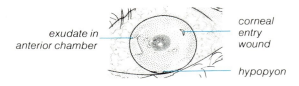

Fig.6.39 Hypopyon uveitis from an intraocular foreign body.

The inflammatory changes do not always occur, and if progressive cataract formation does not take place, the patient may not be aware of the slow deterioration that subsequently occurs from metallosis. This will be discussed in more detail later (see page 9.9).

Preoperative Assessment

Clinical examination

As in all injuries, the initial assessment should start by measuring the visual acuity, and examining the eye for signs of a penetrating injury. Where there is an open eye injury, detailed examination will not be possible. Most patients however have a closed eye injury and careful examination on the slit-lamp will reveal the *portal of entry*. The commonest location is the cornea, but a small subconjunctival haemorrhage at the limbus or over the sclera indicates a more posterior entry.

The size of the entry wound relates to the diameter of the particle; a sealed entry wound (see Fig.6.2) corresponds to a particle size of 2 mm or less, while anything larger will cause a leaking wound and sometimes tissue prolapse.

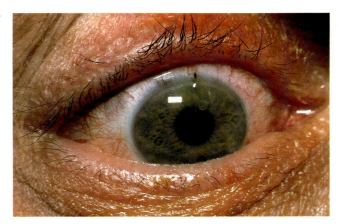

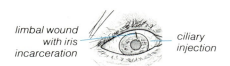

Fig.6.40 Entry wound at the limbus from a large foreign body, showing iris incarceration.

With a corneal entry wound, the direction taken by the foreign body can be predicted from the orientation of the wound. The iris should be examined for signs of damage before dilating the pupil; a hole may be visible in close proximity to the entry wound (seen best by retro-illumination against the red reflex) or the sphincter may be torn.

The pupil should then be dilated with 1% cyclopentolate and 10% phenylephrine to give maximal pupil enlargement; this will allow detailed examination of the lens and subsequent examination of the posterior segment. The foreign body may be visible within the lens, but this is unusual.

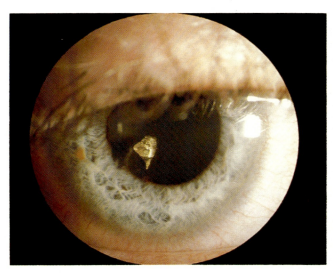

Fig.6.41 Intralenticular foreign body and sphincter tear of the iris.

More commonly the foreign body has passed through the lens. The track may leave little disturbance of the lens cortex, but the site of penetration through both anterior and posterior capsules is clearly visible, particularly when viewed against the red reflex. Small ruptures of the capsule may seal and not lead to progressive changes, but a large rupture will lead to rapid cataract formation.

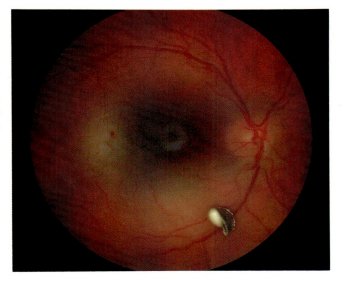

Fig.6.42 Rupture of posterior capsule seen against the red reflex.

An exit wound in the posterior lens capsule confirms that the foreign body has penetrated the posterior segment. In the early stages after injury most foreign bodies can be seen with the indirect ophthalmoscope, even if lens changes are present. This provides the best method of localising a foreign body in the absence of vitreous haemorrhage.

A small foreign body may change direction or lose momentum as it passes through the lens, falling onto the inferior part of the vitreous. It is usually visible near the ora and can be seen with scleral indentation. Larger particles have greater momentum and will traverse the vitreous cavity, ending up by impacting in the retina, or ricocheting to a more anterior location. Vitreous haemorrhage often obscures the position.

Where there is a corneal or limbal entry wound but no sign of lens damage, gonioscopy should be performed as the particle may be located in the drainage angle: this particularly applies to the smallest fragments. If not visible in the angle, the particle may be located in the ciliary body or pars plana.

With a *scleral entry wound,* the particle almost always has sufficient momentum to cross the vitreous cavity and strike the retina. If it impacts in the posterior retina, surrounding retinal oedema and haemorrhage are present (see Fig.6.57). Occasionally it travels further in a subretinal position. If the foreign body rebounds, it may cause retinal damage and its subsequent course may be followed by a track of vitreous haemorrhage (see Fig.6.37). Spasm of a major retinal arteriole can result from local damage leading to loss of central vision.

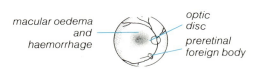

Fig.6.43 Preretinal foreign body with retinal ischaemia from arteriolar damage.

When a posterior ricochet site is visible but no other changes can be seen, the foreign body may have passed through the sclera. It is likely that the particle has perforated the globe for a second time and is no longer within the eye. Accurate localising x-rays or CAT scan will help confirm this.

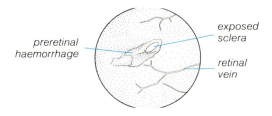

Fig.6.44 Posterior exit wound following double perforation.

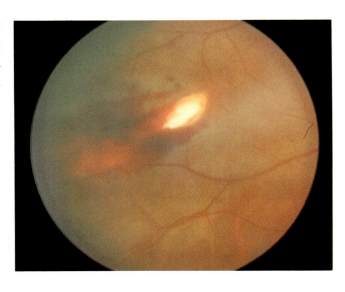

6.19

X-ray examination

All injuries involving the use of a hammer should be x-rayed to exclude a foreign body even if no sign of injury can be detected. Duplicate plain x-rays of the orbit are taken to give two postero-anterior and lateral views; small artefacts may be mistaken for foreign bodies, but will not be present on all films. Hammer injuries give a characteristic boat-shaped particle, while a ragged fragment suggests a non-magnetic material.

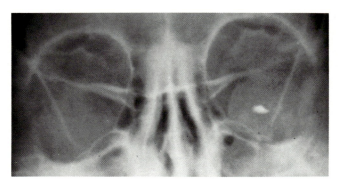

Fig.6.45 X-ray appearance of an intraocular foreign body.

Having confirmed the presence of a metallic intraocular foreign body, its position can be localised with reference to a radio-opaque marker. The Sweet method of positioning a pointer 1cm in front of the eye and taking two exposures (postero-anterior and lateral) was very inaccurate because of eye movement, and has been replaced by a technique involving suturing a sterile stainless steel ring of 12mm diameter around the limbus, or using a sterile suction contact lens containing a radio-opaque ring.

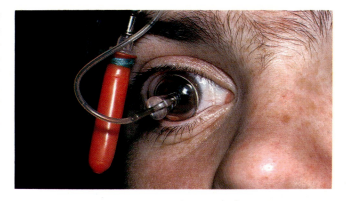

Fig.6.46 Suction contact lens for localising x-rays.

In both cases accurate centration is very important, otherwise errors in localisation will arise. The doctor should check the position of the contact lens during the x-ray examination (note poor centration above) and check the x-rays for correct alignment; a true circle should be seen in the straight films, and a vertical marker in the lateral views.

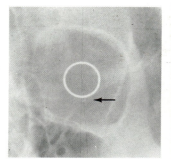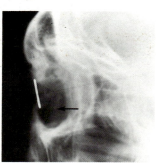

Fig.6.47 left & right Localising ring and foreign body on straight and lateral x-rays.

The postero-anterior x-rays are then marked across the supraorbital margins, and a line is drawn perpendicular to this through the centre of the ring, and obliquely through the ring centre and the foreign body. The angle made by these last two lines is measured and transposed to a plotting chart. A perspex template (Medical Workshop) is centred over the x-ray to give the exact position along this line. Similarly, in the lateral view a line is drawn perpendicular to the centre of the linear mark of the ring, and the antero-posterior position is measured from the template.

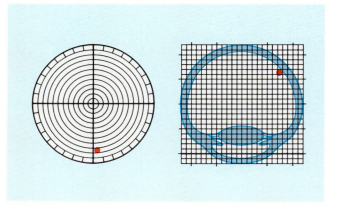

Fig.6.48 Chart showing localisation of a foreign body.

Most difficulty arises with foreign bodies impacted at the posterior pole, where there may be uncertainty as to whether the foreign body is still within the eye. Lateral views taken with the eye in both up- and downgaze are of little value in determining this, as a particle lying just outside the globe will move in a similar fashion to one within the globe.

An alternative method of localisation involves using longitudinal tomography and a set-square marker (G.A.S. Lloyd). This is independent of instrumental contact with the eye and does not depend on accurate placement of a pointer or prolonged co-operation from the patient; accurate longitudinal and vertical measurements can be made. This method is particularly useful for localising multiple intraocular fragments.

Other methods of assessment

The electroacoustic locator provides an invaluable means of locating foreign bodies within the eye; it can be used preoperatively to discriminate between magnetic and non-magnetic particles, and is used during surgery for location of the foreign body. Two types of probe are available for ocular use, which can be sterilised for use during surgery. The straight black probe is more sensitive and is used for detection of particles some distance from the surface, or where the response has become weakened by disintegration of the particle over a period of time. The spatula probe is used most often during surgery; by reducing the sensitivity, the exact point of a foreign body can be marked on the surface of the globe through the central hole in the instrument.

Its use is vital in the removal of small ciliary body or pars plana foreign bodies which cannot be seen (see Fig.6.54), and it is helpful as an additional means of localising foreign bodies in the posterior segment, particularly when the view is obscured by cataract or haemorrhage. It has an additional feature of altering in tone if the particle is external to the probe; this may be helpful in confirming an extraocular position of a foreign body, although it is not always reliable when working far back behind the eye.

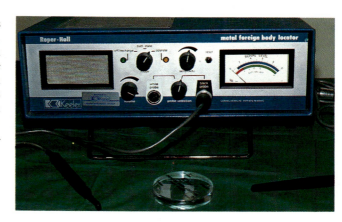

Fig.6.49 The electroacoustic locator, spatula probe (left) and straight black probe (right).

B-scan ultrasonography can help in identifying posterior segment damage and may localise the foreign body, particularly those impacted posteriorly. Similarly, *computerised axial tomography* (CAT scan) can be helpful in confirming whether a small foreign body has emerged posteriorly through the sclera, but with larger fragments too much radiation is reflected for the test to be useful. These investigations will mainly be used prior to secondary surgery for foreign bodies impacted posteriorly.

In some patients a decision may be made not to attempt removal of a steel foreign body; this applies to particles within the lens, or small fragments impacted between the disc and the raphe region, where sugery carries a risk of prejudicing good vision. Dark adaptation, the electro-oculogram and electro-retinogram (see page 7.4) should be monitored every two or three months for the first year, and thereafter at twelve month intervals. Any deterioration in function suggests the onset of siderosis and is an indication for active surgical intervention.

Removal of Magnetic Foreign Bodies

Ideally these foreign bodies should be removed within 24 hours of injury, as a severe inflammatory reaction may rapidly develop. Successful surgery depends on accurate localisation and appropriate facilities for removal. Much harm is caused by injudicious attempts at extraction through the entry wound by 'trial of the magnet'.

With steel particles, the use of an electromagnet through a planned incision is employed to facilitate removal. *Lid sutures* are used instead of a speculum, so that no metal is close to the eye when the electroacoustic locator or magnet is used. These are passed through the drapes and tied, so that the needles can be removed and no forceps are required (see Fig.6.50).

A powerful hand magnet such as the Bronson instrument is often more convenient to use than the giant ring magnet. The magnetic pole of a hand magnet is close to the end of the body, and the short, stubby tips provide a more powerful magnetic field than the long tapering tips. The body of the magnet is enclosed in a sterile plastic bag, and the sterile tips can be screwed through this into the body. During extraction, the magnet should be held perpendicular to the globe surface; brief applications of power should be used, as failure to extract the foreign body immediately implies incorrect localisation, incomplete exposure or too great a distance from the foreign body for the magnet to be effective.

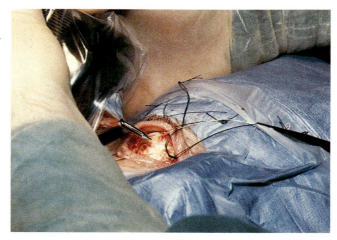

Fig.6.50 Hand magnet in use, protected by a sterile bag.

When removing small particles through an approach that is some distance from the foreign body, or particles that are wealky magnetic, the more powerful giant electromagnet may be required; this is a cumbersome instrument which requires careful positioning so that the affected eye is centred within the ring. A protruding endotracheal tube may interfere with positioning, and the anaesthetist should be warned of this prior to surgery. Soft iron probes held centrally are magnetised by the electromagnetic field; short applications of power should be made, as otherwise the heat generated destroys the magnetism.

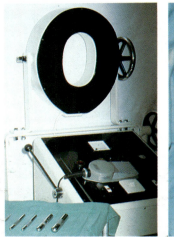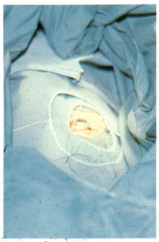

Fig.6.51 left Giant electromagnet.
Fig.6.51 right The electromagnet positioned and draped prior to use.

The Management of Small Intraocular Foreign Bodies

Intraocular foreign bodies of less than 2 mm dimension have a sealed entry wound and no prolapse of tissues. They rarely cause internal haemorrhage, and even if they have passed through the lens, the capsule wounds remain closed and rapid cataract formation does not occur. These injuries should have a good prognosis.

Removal of Anterior Segment Foreign Bodies

Those visible in the anterior segment pose no problem of localisation: the particle may be in the *anterior chamber* (see Fig.6.2) or in the *lens* (see Figs.6.38 and 6.41).

Particles trapped in the *ciliary body* (see Fig.6.39) are more difficult to localise, and the use of the electro-acoustic locator during surgery is of invaluable help.

Foreign bodies in the lens

With intralenticular foreign bodies, if the lens remains clear with good visual function, surgery can be deferred unless retinal function tests (see page 7.4) suggest early iron toxicity. The position of the foreign body will influence this: a completely intralenticular foreign body is in a protected environment and unlikely to cause siderosis; it may be removed with the lens if progressive cataract formation occurs.

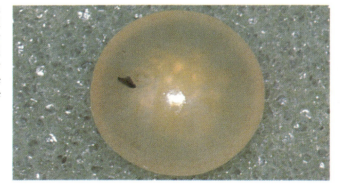

Fig.6.52 Extracted cataract with a foreign body (c f. Fig.6.38 for preoperative appearance).

If the foreign body is protruding through the posterior capsule into the vitreous there is some risk of siderosis (although not great because the retrolental vitreous does not have a high oxygen tension). Surgery is indicated if progressive cataract occurs, or if retinal function tests indicate early siderosis. An intracapsular extraction carries less risk of losing the foreign body into the posterior segment during surgery.

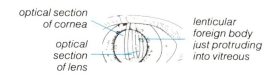

optical section of cornea

optical section of lens

lenticular foreign body just protruding into vitreous

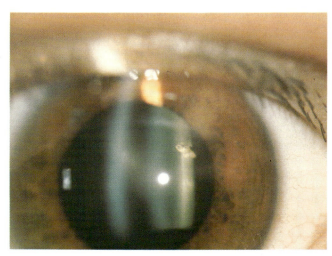

Fig.6.53 Lenticular foreign body protruding into vitreous.

Ciliary body particles

Most particles trapped in the ciliary body will be small; accurate localisation is the secret of success in their removal. If relying on x-ray localisation, the postero-anterior films should be carefully checked to make sure the views are truly straight, otherwise the localised meridian will be wrong. The use of the electroacoustic locator during surgery is particularly helpful in these cases.

1% atropine drops should be instilled before surgery, otherwise muscle spasm may impede removal. The appropriate quadrant of sclera is exposed and traction sutures are placed under the rectus muscle. The position of the foreign body can be confirmed with the electroacoustic locator, and marked on the surface.

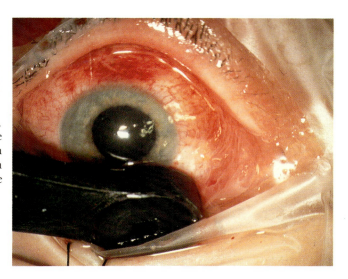

Fig.6.54 Confirming the position of a ciliary body particle using the spatula probe of the electroacoustic locator.

A double trapdoor is then made in the sclera at this point, using bipolar cautery to any bleeding points on the surface of the ciliary body. 0.2 metric (10/0) polypropylene sutures are placed ready for closure of the inner flap, while 0.3 metric (9/0) nylon sutures are preplaced in the outer flap.

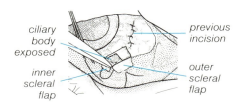

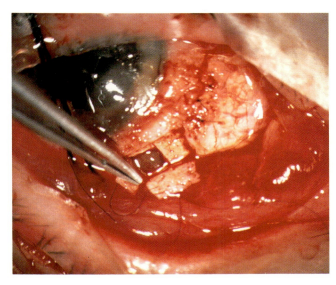

Fig.6.55 Double trapdoor prepared to expose ciliary body (note a previous site of attempted removal based on inaccurate x-ray localisation).

The exposed ciliary body is lifted gently and abscised to perform a small cyclectomy, as the thickness of the tissues in this region may impede the extraction of the foreign body. This is then extracted using a powerful hand magnet or giant electromagnet (see Figs.6.50 and 6.51). If the vitreous prolapses, it should be gently abscised and the wound closed.

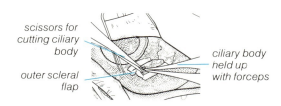

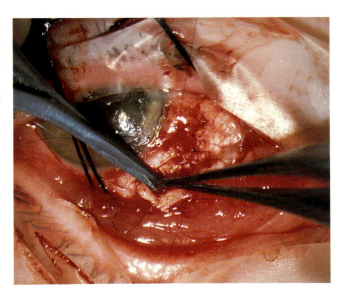

Fig.6.56 Performing a cyclectomy before extracting the foreign body.

If late presentation has led to severe uveitis, a culture should be taken from the extraction site after removal of the foreign body. Full antibiotic treatment should be given, and systemic steroid therapy may be required if rapid resolution does not occur. In most cases the inflammatory reaction is chemical and settles quickly once the foreign body has been removed (the management of intraocular infection is discussed further on page 7.10).

Foreign bodies in the anterior chamber

These will include a few deeply embedded corneal foreign bodies with the tip protruding into the anterior chamber, and those lying on the iris or in the drainage angle; these are usually small fragments. The aim of surgery is to remove these without damaging the lens.

With a deep corneal foreign body the pupil should be constricted prior to surgery. If the foreign body is very deep and at risk of falling into the anterior chamber, a preliminary paracentesis and injection of sodium hyaluronate offers some protection. Anterior removal is easier by slightly enlarging the wound over the foreign body, using a hand magnet for extraction. A minor aqueous leak is expected, but this will seal and suturing is not usually required.

Foreign bodies in the drainage angle are best removed through a scleral flap similar to that raised for a trabeculectomy operation; the position of the foreign body should first be confirmed with the electroacoustic locator or a gonioscope lens. The particle can then be removed with forceps together with a small piece of iris if this is adherent. Iris foreign bodies (see Fig.6.2) can be approached by a more anterior incision and removed with the hand magnet.

Posterior Segment Foreign Bodies: the Management of Small Particles

The particles associated with a closed eye injury are quite small and lose much of their momentum on entering the eye. Some may have sufficient kinetic energy to traverse the globe and impact in the retina posteriorly, while others may ricochet in the pars plana region and spin off into the vitreous. A common location is in the vitreous base region below, particularly with small particles that have traversed the periphery of the lens. These small particles are rarely associated with vitreous haemorrhage.

The surgical options:

1. Direct magnetic removal through the closest point.

2. Indirect magnetic removal via a pars plana incision.

3. Transvitreal removal with instrumentation.

The surgical approach

With a fresh injury, if a small foreign body is impacted in the retina or lying very close to it, the simplest approach is *direct removal* through the overlying tissues if it can be reached. This may necessitate detaching a rectus muscle. With this approach, the foreign body can be accurately localised both with the indirect ophthalmoscope and the electroacoustic locator; magnetic extraction is facilitated by close proximity to the particle. In fresh injuries, the particle is sharp and will come cleanly through the retina without incarceration.

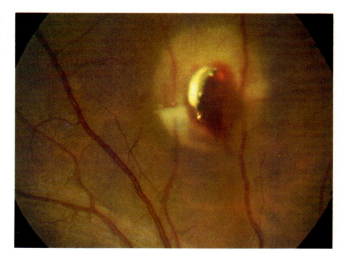

Fig.6.57 Impacted foreign body suitable for direct removal.

If a small particle is floating freely in the posterior vitreous, or impacted close to the optic disc or macula, a direct approach cannot be used, and pars plana extraction is unlikely to be successful because of the distance between the particle and the magnet. In this situation transvitreal removal is carried out (see page 9.6). The same technique should also be considered for any preretinal foreign body where removal has been delayed, as fibrosis around the particle causes retinal adhesion which may lead to retinal incarceration if direct removal is attempted.

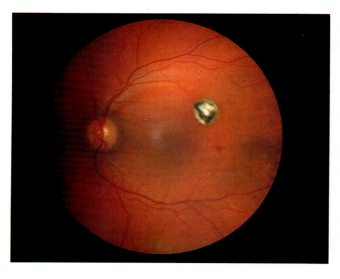

Fig.6.58 Particle lying close to the macula needing transvitreal removal.

Direct removal

The first step is to confirm the position of the foreign body using the indirect ophthalmoscope and scleral indentation. The position is marked on the surface with a suture and confirmed by further inspection. Cryotherapy is performed where the foreign body is lying in the vitreous, but is probably not needed for impacted foreign bodies, as the local contusion stimulates pigment hyperplasia and adhesion. The electroacoustic locator can also be used to pinpoint the foreign body and confirm its magnetic nature.

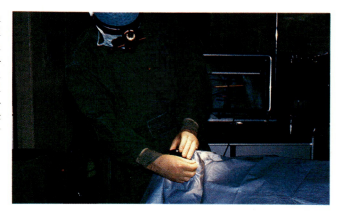

Fig.6.59 Localisation using the indirect ophthalmoscope.

Although it is common practice to raise a scleral flap and remove the foreign body through an incision in the deep lamella of sclera, this technique is likely to give complications from tissue prolapse. It is better to perform a simple linear full-thickness scleral incision; the underlying choroid and retina are not incised in fresh injuries as these foreign bodies are sharp and will come cleanly through the incision using a powerful electromagnet.

In this illustration a scleral flap has been raised and a linear incision is being made in the deep lamella.

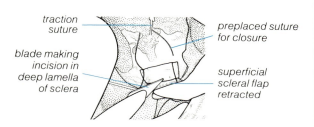

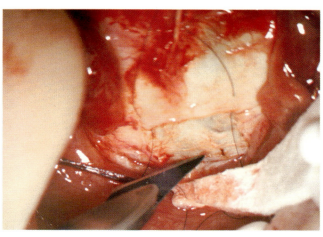

Fig.6.60 Linear incision through the deeper layer of sclera after raising a flap.

Removal is carried out with the hand magnet; if the foreign body is not extracted after one or two applications, it will be because of inaccurate localisation, an incision too small or incomplete, or because the particle is non-magnetic. If localisation is correct and the particle is known to be magnetic, the scleral incision should be slightly enlarged before applying the magnet again. The entry wound is a useful guide to the size of sclerotomy required for removal of the foreign body.

In this example, the foreign body has been extracted without difficulty but the thinness of the deep scleral lamella has allowed bulging of tissues through the wound with a greater risk of incarceration. This is avoided by a simple full-thickness sclerotomy.

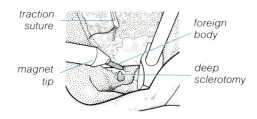

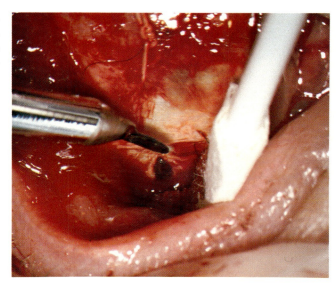

Fig.6.61 Magnetic removal of the foreign body. Note bulging of tissues through the thin sclerotomy.

6.25

After closing the sclerotomy, an important part of the operation is examining the fundus with the indirect ophthalmoscope; the site of extraction is inspected to see that no retinal incarceration is present. If there is any evidence of this, the wound should be revised; if incarceration persists, sodium hyaluronate is injected gently into the lips of the wound. The presence of internal haemorrhage should be recorded, as visibility may decrease in the postoperative period from lens opacities. This information is important; if a haemorrhagic track or diffuse vitreous haemorrhage is present, vitrectomy will be indicated later.

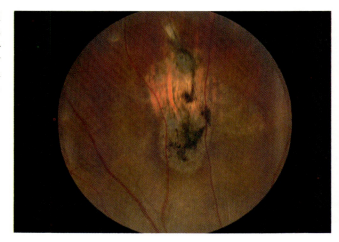

If required, cryotherapy is best applied before removal of the foreign body, as any manipulation afterwards may precipitate bleeding. A small preretinal haemorrhage may occur, but this usually clears without any complications. Local indentation is not necessary in fresh foreign bodies removed through the retina, but is essential after removal of retained particles (page 9.11).

Fig.6.62 Later view of the extraction site after direct removal and cryotherapy (c f. Fig.6.57).

Transvitreal removal

A small foreign body in the vitreous or impacted at the posterior pole cannot be removed by a direct approach, and transvitreal surgery will be necessary (see page 9.6). Those free in the vitreous will need early removal, but those impacted in the retina, particularly if very close to the macula (see Fig.6.58), may be observed for a period before embarking on surgery. Many impacted foreign bodies will encapsulate, and conservative management may be less traumatic than attempted removal.

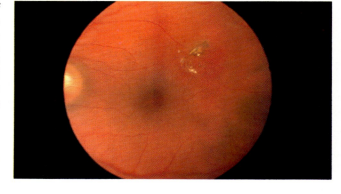

Fig.6.63 Appearance of the retina after transvitreal removal of a foreign body embedded near the macula (c f. Fig.6.58).

If the particle is not removed, a ring of laser treatment to create an avascular scar around the foreign body may help prevent siderosis; electrodiagnostic tests should be monitored as discussed earlier (see page 6.21).

The Management of Large Particles

These large intraocular foreign bodies are associated with an open wound with tissue prolapse, and with extensive internal damage. *These fragments have a high kinetic energy and always strike the back of the eye.* They may impact posteriorly or even perforate the globe for a second time, and are often obscured by preretinal haemorrhage (see Fig.6.37). The particle may rebound to end up in the equatorial region; diffuse vitreous haemorrhage from the ricochet site is common, preventing an adequate view of the foreign body.

The surgical approach

The entry wound and related damage will require repair as described for perforating eye injuries; this includes wound toilet and watertight closure, followed by lensectomy and anterior vitrectomy if the lens has been disrupted. Where facilities for this are not available, surgery should be limited to wound toilet and closure, and the patient should be referred to a specialist centre.

The same surgical options (see page 6.24) are available for removing the foreign body as described for small particles, but planning the removal is complicated by the presence of internal haemorrhage which may obscure the exact location of the foreign body. If visible and impacted in an accessible site, direct removal is carried out (although if the particle has been retained for a few days transvitreal removal is better, as discussed on page 6.24). If the particle is lying free in the vitreous or the view is obscured by haemorrhage, a pars plana approach is carried out.

These larger particles can be attracted by the electro-magnet over a much greater distance. A generous linear incision should be made in the sclera 4–5 mm behind the limbus. After cauterising the uveal tissue an incision is made in it which may need extending with fine scissors to ensure a large enough opening is present. After removing the foreign body any prolapsed tissue should be meticulously excised to avoid incarceration, otherwise vitreous base traction may occur leading to retinal detachment.

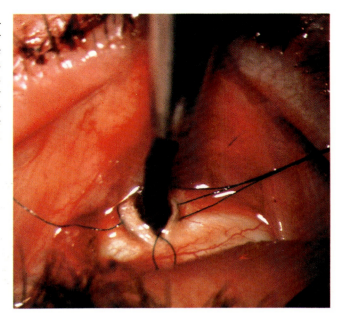

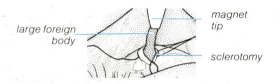

Fig.6.64 Removal of a large intraocular foreign body via a pars plana incision.

If the intraocular body is impacted posteriorly and attempted removal via the pars plana fails, a further attempt at removal should be deferred and undertaken as a secondary procedure together with a pars plana vitrectomy. Unless an acute inflammatory reaction develops, this is best planned two to four weeks after injury to reduce the risk of secondary haemorrhage and to allow the posterior vitreous to detach completely. Some of these particles have perforated the globe poster-iorly and are no longer intraocular; it is important not to make repeated attempts to extract the particle and cause additional trauma to the eye.

Particles of this size will have caused retinal damage by internal ricochet, and most of these will have a haemor-rhagic track to the extraction site or diffuse vitreous haemorrhage. This will lead to secondary fibrosis and traction bands to the site of retinal damage which, if untreated, will lead to retinal detachment (see Fig.6.70). All patients with an entry wound that requires suturing will need to be considered for secondary vitrectomy. This is discussed in more detail later (see page 9.5).

Non-Magnetic Intraocular Foreign Bodies

The *history* is very important in these injuries for identifying the nature of the foreign body. These injuries usually result from some form of explosion or from a ballistic missile. In some cases the true history is not given (particularly in children). A common injury arises from hammering an explosive cartridge, but is often repre-sented as hammering a stone; the x-ray appearance should be inspected to see if it is consistent with a steel fragment from a hammer injury. A ragged fragment should always suggest a non-magnetic particle.

Explosive injuries involving castings may result in metal fragments such as aluminium penetrating the eye. The x-ray appearance may be deceptive, as these particles are relatively radiolucent.

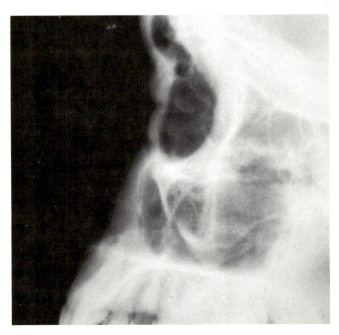

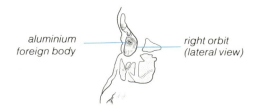

Fig.6.65 X-ray appearance of aluminium within the right eye.

Copper-based foreign bodies usually cause a violent endophthalmitis within hours of injury and vitreous surgery may need to be carried out as an emergency procedure; in injuries with posterior segment damage, secondary bleeding is common which may hamper visibility and prevent removal of the particle. Lead and aluminium are less toxic to the eye; in these cases the primary surgery should be confined to wound toilet and repair, and removal of the foreign body carried out as a secondary procedure when the risk of secondary bleeding has diminished.

Removal of a non-magnetic foreign body requires direct instrumentation within the eye using vitrectomy techniques (see page 9.7).

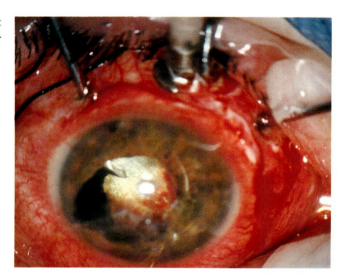

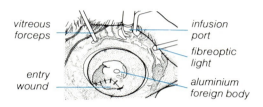

Fig.6.66 Large fragment of aluminium held by vitreous forceps prior to anterior removal.

Some of these injuries are due to air-gun pellets that have ricocheted and flattened to give a sharp edge; double perforation in this group is common. After cleaning and repairing the entry wound, the posterior aspect of the globe should be examined for an exit wound, and the pellet may be found close to this. If it is intraocular, removal should not be attempted at primary repair as it is relatively inert, and more harm than good is done by instrumentation within the eye at this stage.

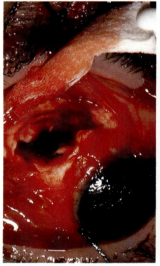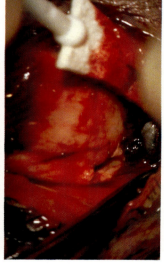

Fig.6.67 left Anterior entry wound of air-gun pellet.
Fig.6.67 right Posterior exit wound with pellet outside the globe.

These injuries have extensive intraocular damage, with major internal bleeding; often there is no light perception prior to repair, and many of these cases end up being enucleated.

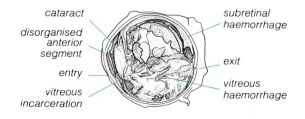

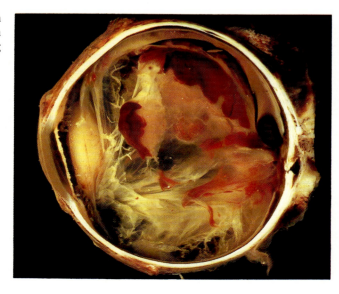

Fig.6.68 Section of an enucleated eye after double perforation from a shot-gun pellet. By courtesy of Prof. W.R. Lee.

After successfully removing any foreign body, its size and shape should be recorded and the particle filed for reference purposes. Many of these injuries will be the subject of a medicolegal claim, and the particle will need to be available for examination.

The postoperative management is similar to that for perforating eye injuries (see page 6.10); both topical and systemic antibiotics are given, plus cycloplegic and local steroid drops. Tetanus prophylaxis is also required. Patients with posterior segment damage should be kept on bed rest for a few days to minimise the risk of secondary haemorrhage. When mobile, the patient should be *x-rayed again* to confirm that the foreign body has been removed.

The management of lens damage

A track from a small particle does not necessarily result in progressive cataract formation: many of these will remain as localised lens opacities with good preservation of vision. In others, slow development of cataract occurs, and this can be dealt with by conventional surgery at a later date. The cataract should be removed *before* it has become mature, otherwise lens swelling may lead to rupture through the weakened point in the capsule. Intracapsular surgery is the method of choice in the older age group, as the posterior capsule may give way during conventional extracapsular surgery; an intraocular lens should not be inserted if the injury has caused posterior segment damage. In the younger age group lensectomy is the treatment of choice.

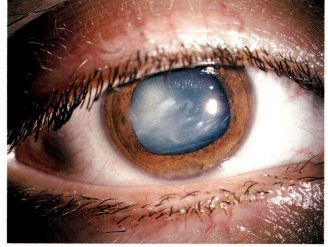

Fig.6.69 Rapid maturation of a traumatic cataract after an intraocular foreign body.

A large hole in either the anterior or posterior capsule will not seal, and leads to rapid lens swelling. Anterior rupture is more common than posterior, but rapid maturation of a cataract and increasing uveitis with an apparently intact anterior surface suggests rupture into the vitreous.

Ultrasonography can confirm the reaction present behind the lens (see page 7.3). Most of these injuries will have sustained significant posterior segment damage, and lensectomy is best performed as part of a planned pars plana vitrectomy (see page 8.5).

The management of posterior segment damage

The preoperative assessment and any changes observed at completion of surgery are very important in the subsequent management, as a decision on further treatment may need to be based on these findings. *Any patient with either a haemorrhagic track crossing the vitreous or diffuse vitreous haemorrhage plus an area of retinal damage will need vitrectomy.* Localised preretinal haemorrhage does not require vitrectomy, and can be observed. The extraction site should be checked for any signs of incarceration; this is important if a pars plana approach has been used, as traction on the vitreous base may lead to retinal breaks and subsequent detachment.

Before vitreous surgery became available, 33% of fresh intraocular foreign bodies lost all useful vision. Some of these injuries (8%) represented those damaged beyond repair; in 25% the early outcome was encouraging, but vision was lost later because of traction retinal detachment. Conventional surgery was usually unsuccessful in correcting this.

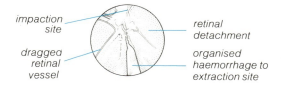

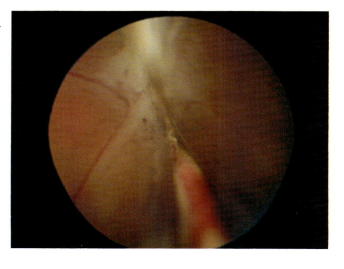

Fig.6.70 Established traction detachment after pars plana removal of an intraocular foreign body.

With vitrectomy techniques, the incidence of retinal detachment has fallen dramatically; the acuity however is often disappointing, as many of these injuries have damaged the posterior pole, and macular pucker is common. This subject is discussed in more detail in Chapter 9.

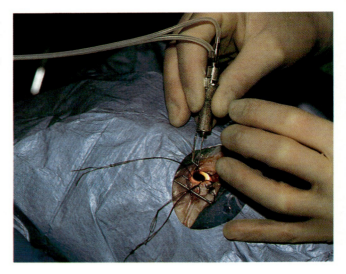

Fig.6.71 Vitrectomy following posterior segment damage, using the indirect ophthalmoscope.

Retained intraocular foreign bodies
This term should be reserved for those patients presenting with the late complications of a metallic foreign body within the eye.

The clinical presentation and management of these injuries is discussed on page 9.5.

7

The Management of Complicated Injuries: Introduction

ASSESSMENT OF THE BADLY INJURED EYE

In severe injuries, the full extent of intraocular damage is initially obscured by internal bleeding or opacities in the media; before planning surgery for complications such as cataract or vitreous haemorrhage, a period of assessment is needed to evaluate the extent of damage and the visual potential.

Clinical Assessment

The assessment on presentation will give valuable information that will help predict complications; this has been described in detail in the earlier chapters. The subsequent progress needs careful monitoring, and assessment should include symptoms such as pain and photophobia, the level of vision and the clinical findings.

Increasing pain always indicates serious pathology: an abrupt onset accompanies internal bleeding, such as recurrent hyphaema or a suprachoroidal haemorrhage, but a slower onset of pain accompanies a rise of intraocular pressure, increasing uveitis, or intraocular infection. Most injured eyes are initially photophobic, but this should improve. To assess this, the eye should be uncovered but protected with dark glasses.

Regular assessment of vision is important; in severe injuries, vision may be reduced to light perception only, and projection of light should be tested in a darkened room. Eyes with absent light perception or grossly defective light projection have a poor prognosis, because of disruption of the vital structures in the posterior segment. These injured eyes usually follow a downhill course, but occasionally improvement occurs.

Uveitis is present to some extent in all injuries: the degree of ciliary injection and anterior chamber activity should be monitored, and the level of intraocular pressure recorded. Increasing aqueous flare and hypotony are unfavourable signs, which may be a warning of sympathetic ophthalmitis (see page 7.11).

The structural changes encountered after the various types of injury have been discussed in earlier chapters. In many cases visibility will be impaired by opacities in the media, and other methods of assessment are required. Ultrasonography helps to assess structural changes while electrodiagnostic tests assess retinal function. The combined evaluation of these tests provides a better assessment than either test alone.

Assessment of Injured Eyes with Opaque Media

Ultrasonography
This technique sends short pulses of high frequency sound into the eye via a transducer. Echoes reflected from tissue interfaces are detected by the same transducer and are amplified and displayed on a screen as an ultrasonogram. The amplitude of the echoes reflects the density of the tissue interface and this can be quantitated by the A-scan technique (single dimension). B-scan techniques (two-dimensional) provide a display of the globe in section, and repeated scans can be taken from different directions.

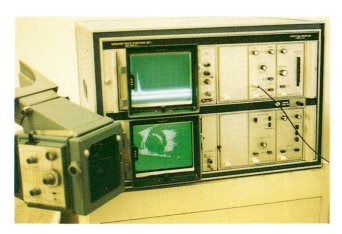

Fig.7.1 A-and B-scans displayed.

A water–bath technique allows better definition of anterior segment structures and permits dynamic studies, which are helpful in assessing mechanical damage within the eye. In some machines the water–bath is incorporated into the transducer, allowing scanning through the closed eyelids; this is an advantage when scanning recently traumatised eyes.

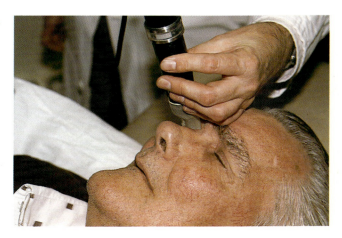

Fig.7.2 B-scan ultrasonography using the Ocuscan transducer.

This technique can demonstrate a variety of pathological changes resulting from injury: changes in lens position can be identified from its characteristic biconvex shape, while cataractous change shows up as an increasing density of the lens echoes.

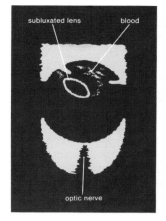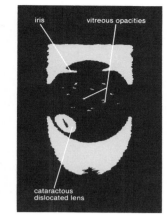

Fig.7.3 USG appearance of a clear subluxated lens (left) and a posteriorly dislocated cataractous lens (right).

A posterior rupture of the lens can occur after the passage of an intraocular foreign body; it is suggested by a cone of soft echoes in the vitreous behind a cataract. Continued inflammation may lead to a cyclitic membrane, which is seen as a rigid opacity behind the iris.

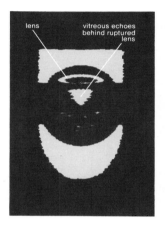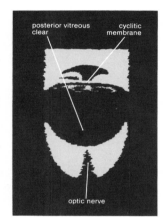

Fig.7.4 USG appearance of a posterior rupture of a lens (left) and a cyclitic membrane (right).

Intragel vitreous haemorrhage initially shows widespread low-amplitude echoes, but after separation of the vitreous from the retina (see page 7.6) the posterior hyaloid surface produces a discrete interface that remains mobile. By contrast, vitreous haemorrhage associated with a penetrating wound leads to an organised posterior hyaloid, resulting in a rigid funnel to a point of retinal damage. This can be confused with a fibrotic retinal detachment, but the latter always originates from the optic disc.

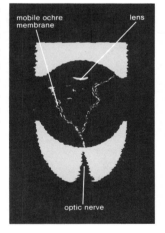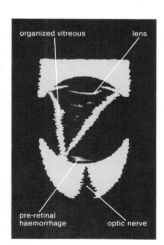

Fig.7.5 USG appearance of an ochre membrane (left) and a rigid vitreous fibrosis to a point of retinal damage from an intraocular foreign body (right).

After major ocular trauma, suprachoroidal, subretinal and preretinal haemorrhages are common. Large suprachoroidal haemorrhages may initially give solid echoes, but the blood subsequently liquefies to give silent convexities that protrude into the cavity. Subretinal and preretinal haemorrhages remain as dense opacities for some time. Early retinal separation produces a shallow elevation that terminates at the optic disc, although in time an extensive funnel detachment may form.

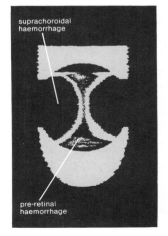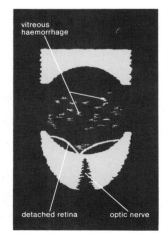

Fig.7.6 USG appearance of large, old suprachoroidal and preretinal haemorrhage (left) and a diffuse vitreous haemorrhage and shallow retinal detachment (right).

Electrodiagnostic tests

The *electro-oculogram* measures the resting potential generated by the pigment epithelium of the retina. As the eye moves between two surface electrodes, a change in potential is recorded while the retina moves nearer or further from the active lead. The response is less when dark-adapted than when light-adapted, and the result is recorded as a ratio of the two values and compared with the norm of test conditions. The electro-oculogram will be affected in conditions that damage the pigment epithelium, and is important in the early detection of siderosis (see page 9.10).

The *electroretinogram* (ERG) measures the change in the electrical potential generated in the retina in response to a light stimulus, and provides an overall assessment of retinal function. The normal technique uses a contact lens electrode, but this is often unsuitable after major trauma; in this situation, a gold-leaf electrode resting on the cornea is used as the active lead, with a reference electrode at the outer canthus.

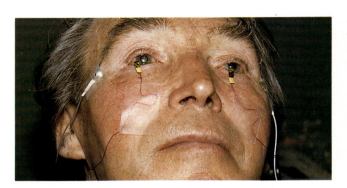

Fig.7.7 Electrode placement for skin electroretinography.

The responses to repeated photostimulation from a Grass stroboscope are averaged by a digital analyser and then recorded. The amplitude of the B-wave is used to measure retinal function. If this is less than 50% normal, the prognosis for vision is poor. Significant opacities in the media may prevent adequate stimulus of the retina when using the conventional stroboscope. Cataract alone does not reduce the electroretinogram, but dense vitreous haemorrhage may affect the result. A bright flash technique can overcome this and result in an improvement in the recorded electroretinogram.

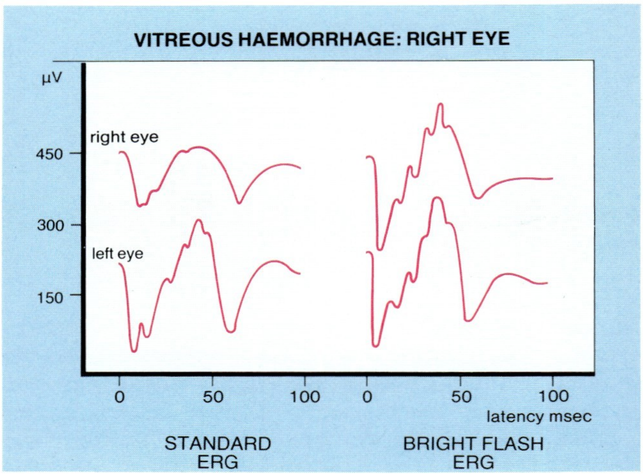

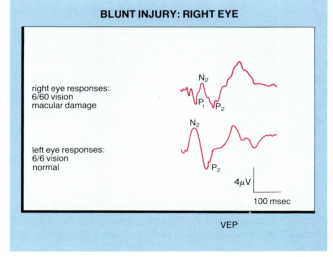

Fig.7.8 A reduced ERG in the right eye with dense vitreous haemorrhage and a retained steel particle, improving with the bright flash technique.

The electroretinogram will reflect any changes that interfere with retinal function. It is temporarily impaired after a concussion injury, while any injury that leads to retinal detachment will reduce the response in proportion to the area affected. Displacement by suprachoroidal haemorrhage also reduces the response by preventing adequate stimulation of the receptors. The electroretinogram is severely reduced by siderosis and will ultimately be extinguished. Together with the electro-oculogram, the electroretinogram is important in the management of retained intraocular foreign bodies (see page 9.10).

The *Visual Evoked Potential* (VEP) reflects damage to the macula or the higher visual pathways. In a major eye injury vision is often too poor to test pattern responses, and a flash response to a Grass stroboscope is recorded. Scalp electrodes are placed over each occiput and referred to right and left central electrodes. The amplitude and latency of the P2 component of the response is measured and expressed as a percentage of the uninjured eye or of the age-matched norm when both eyes have been injured. A reduction of the P2 component that exceeds 50% or is delayed beyond 30 msec carries a poor prognosis for central vision.

Fig.7.9 A reduced and delayed VEP after blunt trauma to the right eye with macular damage, compared with the normal response from the other eye.

7.4

Removal of an Injured Eye

After a penetrating trauma, a decision needs to be made within the first two weeks as to whether the eye is safe to retain; the visual and cosmetic potential of the injured eye must be weighed against the risk of sympathetic ophthalmitis (see page 7.11). Our policy is to remove any perforated eye that has no light perception or inaccurate light projection and is becoming phthisical.

Some injured eyes with a full hyphaema and doubtful light projection may slowly improve, with recovery of intraocular pressure and reformation of the anterior chamber. Unless these eyes are irritable, they may be observed for a longer period to see if further improvement occurs.

Any injured eye that continues to be irritable despite treatment should be considered for enucleation. Although modern surgery has helped prevent the blinding consequences of intraocular fibrosis, multiple operations may carry a higher risk of sympathetic ophthalmitis.

Enucleation

Removing a recently injured eye may be difficult because of bleeding from congested vessels and multiple adhesions. An orbital implant will reduce the socket volume and assist the movement of the prosthesis. If a magnet is incorporated to the implant and subsequent prosthesis, movement of the artificial eye will be greatly enhanced.

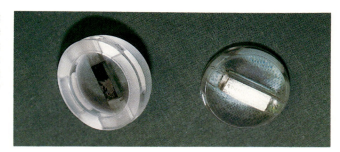

Fig.7.10 Magnetic orbital implant.

Evisceration

When gross intraocular infection is present, evisceration rather than enucleation is performed to prevent spread of bacteria to the meninges. This procedure is also occasionally performed during primary surgery for a severe penetrating injury with tissue loss and expulsion of intraocular contents, where it is clear that no visual or cosmetic recovery can be expected.

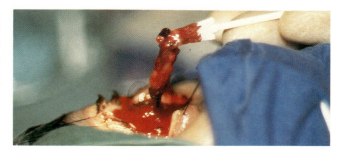

Fig.7.11 Retinal prolapse identified prior to evisceration of a severe perforating injury.

The Management of an Unsightly, Blind Eye

If an injured eye is not removed at an early stage and becomes blind and disorganized, it is likely to shrink and become cosmetically unacceptable. A divergent squint also commonly develops.

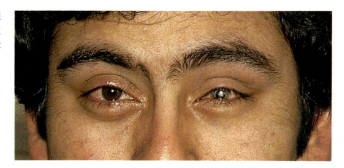

Fig.7.12 An unsightly phthisical eye after trauma.

If the eye is comfortable, a good cosmetic result can be achieved with a haptic contact lens painted to match the other eye, although marked divergence of the affected eye can make fitting impracticable. If a contact lens is not tolerated, enucleation can be offered.

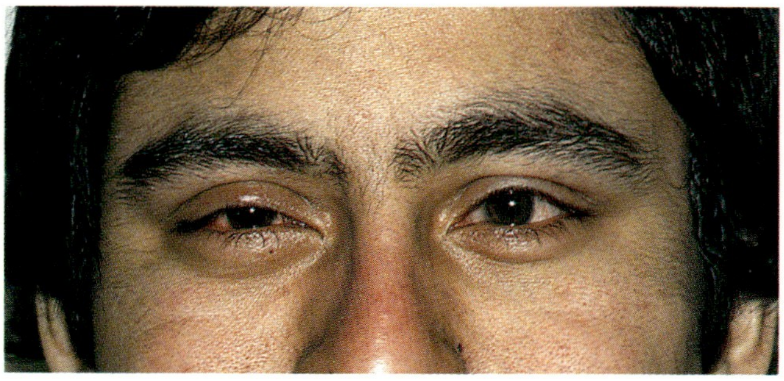

Fig.7.13 Improved appearance with a cosmetic contact lens.

Tissue damage resulting in vitreous haemorrhage is the major stimulus to intraocular fibrosis after an eye injury. Lens damage contributes by increasing the inflammatory reaction. An understanding of the patho-logical changes that follow a simple vitreous haemorrhage and the influence of a penetrating wound is helpful in planning the subsequent management.

Vitreous Haemorrhage without Perforation

Intragel haemorrhage

The immediate effect of a dense intragel haemorrhage is clot formation, followed by fibrinolysis and depolymerisation of hyaluronic acid, leading to collapse of the collagen framework. Gel separation from the posterior retina occurs about six days later, and is often followed by collapse of the gel structure; this can remain attached to the optic disc forming a funnel, or separate completely and remain in the equatorial plane. Attachments persist to sites of abnormal vitreoretinal adhesion. In young patients gel separation takes longer.

Ochre membrane

The erythrocytes undergo slow haemolysis leaving 'ghost cells' (erythroclasts) that become compacted against the detached posterior vitreous face and on the vitreous fibrils; this results in a dense opacity that has a yellow tinge named 'ochre membrane'.

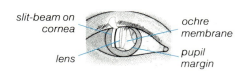

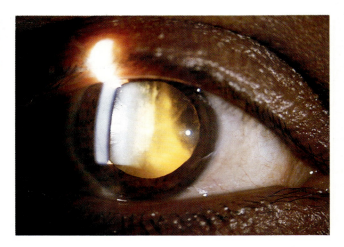

Fig.7.14 'Ochre membrane' following an intragel vitreous haemorrhage.

Vitreous Pathology after a Penetrating Wound

Scleral laceration without vitreous haemorrhage

If incarceration of tissues is avoided and there is no vitreous haemorrhage, fibrovascular proliferation is limited to the wound area. Loss of vitreous leads to gel separation from the retina, but the detached posterior vitreous face remains mobile. If incarcerated vitreous cortex is left in the wound, traction to the adjacent vitreous base is present from the outset. The incarceration stimulates fibroplasia along the surface of the retina and the retrohyaloid face, resulting in progressive traction and retinal detachment.

Scleral laceration with vitreous haemorrhage

With anterior scleral lacerations and localised vitreous haemorrhage, limited fibroproliferation occurs along adjacent surfaces, extending over the ciliary body and onto the posterior surface of the lens, or tangentially in the vitreous base region. Ultimately, traction on the vitreous base causes a localised peripheral retinal detachment, which slowly progresses.

With diffuse vitreous haemorrhage rapid organisation of the vitreous occurs, with traction on the vitreous base. If untreated, these injuries all progress to total retinal detachment.

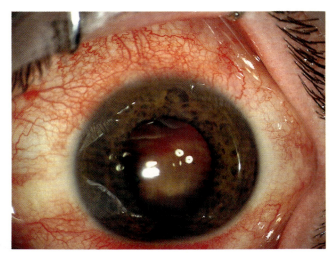

Fig.7.15 Diffuse vitreous haemorrhage becoming organised after an inferior scleral laceration.

Dense vitreous haemorrhage usually complicates large posterior segment intraocular foreign bodies. Rapid fibroplasia develops which extends onto the surface of the retina, the retrohyaloid face and along haemorrhagic tracks to the sites of retinal damage.

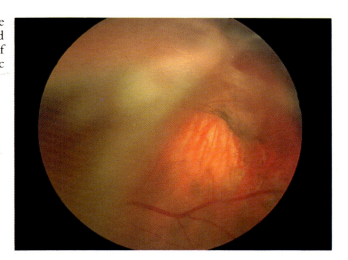

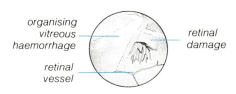

Fig.7.16 Organising vitreous haemorrhage following an intraocular foreign body.

Lens damage with vitreous haemorrhage

In extensive corneo-scleral perforations, the expulsion of iris, lens and vitreous leaves little scaffold for intra-ocular fibrosis. In less severe injuries, damaged lens matter mixed with vitreous haemorrhage results in a severe inflammatory reaction and fibroplasia leading to a cyclitic membrane, hypotony, and ultimately to retinal detachment.

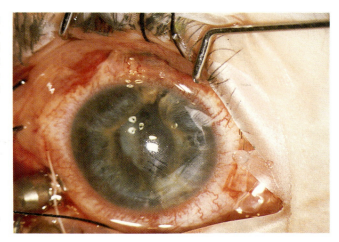

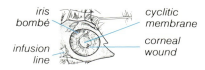

Fig.7.17 Cyclitic membrane from anterior segment fibrosis after a dart injury.

The rate of development of fibroplasia

This depends on the extent of tissue damage and will occur more quickly in eyes with dense vitreous haemorrhage and marked inflammation. In experimental studies, the early inflammatory and proliferative responses are confined to the wound area, but after three days macrophages migrate into the vitreous and cellular proliferation commences. The inflammatory changes are maximal at fourteen days, but fibroplasia develops more slowly, reaching a peak four to six weeks after injury.

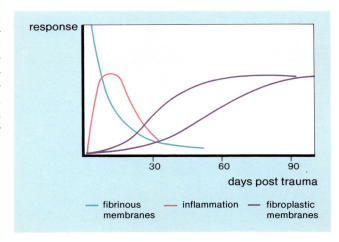

Fig.7.18 Diagram showing the rate of fibroplasia after penetrating trauma.

The Timing of Secondary Surgery

Removing damaged tissues from an injured eye reduces the stimulus to intraocular fibrosis and helps prevent some of the blinding complications. Anterior segment damage should be dealt with at primary repair; the importance of adequate removal of a damaged lens mixed with vitreous has already been emphasised (see page 6.14).

In posterior segment injuries with vitreous haemor-rhage, an interval of one week allows separation of the vitreous from the posterior retina, which makes vitrec-tomy safer. In injuries associated with an element of contusion, a longer interval is required before surgery because of the risk of recurrent bleeding. Secondary surgery is usually carried out two to six weeks after injury.

In the subsequent sections reference will be made to closed microsurgical techniques for dealing with anterior or posterior segment complications. The general principles and basic technique are outlined here, while further details required for specific problems will be discussed in Chapters 8 and 9.

Our experience has mainly been with the Ocutome

vitreous cutter: the vitrectomy probe has a side opening near the tip through which damaged tissue is aspirated under controlled suction; internally the pneumatically-driven guillotine-cutter abscises and removes the aspirated material. The port size, suction pressure and cutting rate can be varied, and the machine stops with the port open.

Current systems are based on standard 20-gauge incisions or 'ports', and all the various instruments used (including intraocular scissors, forceps etc.) are of the same size to give a watertight seal when in use. Infusion of a balanced salt solution maintains the intraocular pressure while the procedure is carried out, and internal bleeding during surgery is controlled by using the intraocular bipolar cautery.

A cutter	**F** cupped forceps
B scleral plugs	**G** vitreous scissors
C contact lens	**H** vitreous forceps
D flute needle	**I** bipolar probe
E fibreoptic light	**J** infusion needle and tubing

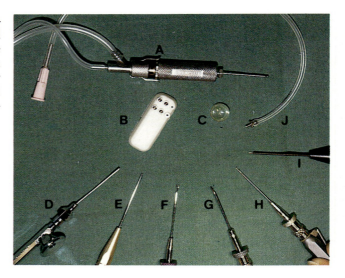

Fig.7.19 Various 20-gauge instruments for use in closed microsurgery.

Anterior Surgery

Two corneal or limbal incisions are made with a standard 20-gauge blade, and peripheral iridectomies are performed. Infusion is via a blunt 20-gauge needle, and the cutter is used at a slow speed and high suction. This approach is used for removing hyphaema or a damaged lens; the cutting mode is used to remove capsule or clotted blood, while soft lens matter can be aspirated. The manipulations are viewed through the coaxially illuminated operating microscope.

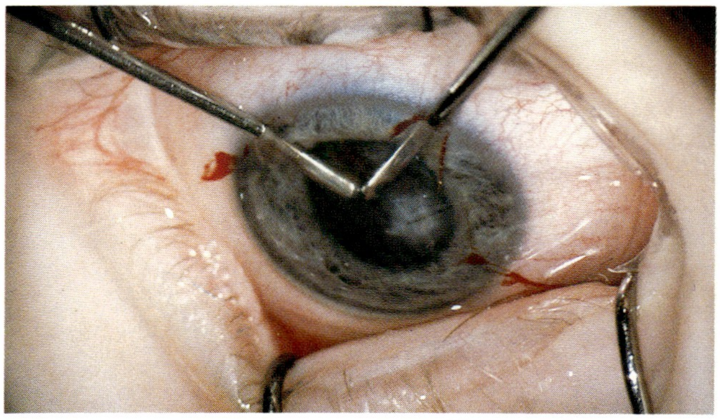

Fig.7.20 The bimanual technique for anterior closed microsurgery.

A limited anterior vitrectomy can be performed from this approach in aphakic eyes but if more extensive surgery is required, a pars plana approach is preferred. An infusion line is secured (see Fig. 7.22), leaving both hands free for using other instruments. The infusion needles are available in different lengths, ranging from 2.5 to 6.0 mm; the shorter length is preferred in normotensive, phakic eyes, but the longer length is used in soft eyes to ensure entering the vitreous cavity.

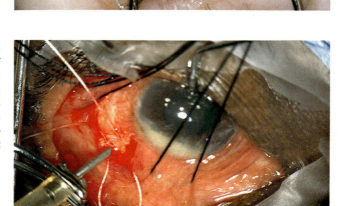

Fig.7.21 The 6 mm infusion needle being inserted in an aphakic eye with endophthalmitis.

This approach is used for procedures such as removal of a subluxated lens or a cyclitic membrane (see pages 8.9 and 8.11), where tissue needs to be removed from behind the pupil. Access to the anterior chamber is possible in the aphakic eye for removal of organised exudate and separation of synechiae (see Fig.7.26).

The first step is to insert traction sutures under the appropriate rectus muscles and expose the sclera. If an encirclement is planned, the band is sutured in position before proceeding.

The infusion line is usually set up in the lower temporal quadrant, but if this is involved in the pathology, an alternative site (usually higher up) is chosen. A sterile drip-line is connected up to the infusion needle after moving the on-off control near to the outlet, so that the assistant can adjust this during surgery.

Episcleral vessels are cauterised, and a mattress suture (1.0 metric (5/0) braided polyester) is positioned 3.5 mm behind the limbus. A standard 20-gauge blade is introduced radially well into the vitreous cavity, and the opening is dilated with a 19-gauge needle. The infusion needle is inserted into the sclerotomy using a screw-action, with the infusion turned half on. The mattress suture is then secured and the infusion is opened fully.

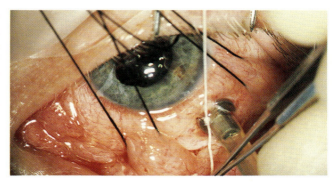

Fig.7.22 Securing the infusion needle.

Similar sclerotomies are then prepared at the two and ten o' clock positions if the vitrectomy is being performed under microscopic control. The cutter needs priming with sterile saline to expel the air from the system before it is introduced into the eye. All foot controls are checked and the microscope is focused at the top of its range. The instruments are introduced obliquely downwards and centrally until visible through the pupil.

For posterior vitrectomy, the contact lens is positioned on the cornea. The internal manoeuvres are illuminated by the fibreoptic probe with the microscope light off, leaving the focusing and zoom functions operational. The size of the cutting port and the level of suction are reduced when working near the retina, and the cutting rate is increased to around 400/min.

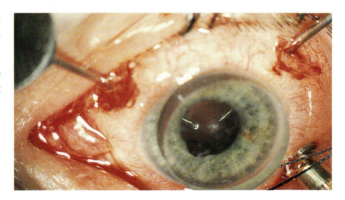

Fig.7.23 Cutter and fibreoptic light visible in the anterior vitreous through the contact lens.

At the end of the procedure the infusion is turned off before removing the instruments from the eye, otherwise tissue will prolapse into the sclerotomies. These are cleaned and closed with 0.3 metric (9/0) nylon, before completing any retinal surgery. Subconjunctival and systemic antibiotics are given routinely, together with subconjunctival betamethasone 4 mg and topical atropine.

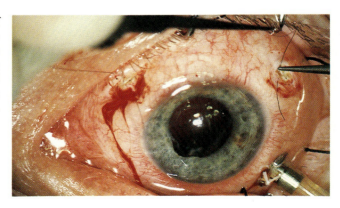

Fig.7.24 Closure of the sclerotomies at the end of the procedure.

The vitreous cutter cannot aspirate tough fibrous sheets or thick bands, and these need to be incised and cut with intraocular scissors (see Fig.7.19) prior to removing with the cutter.

Access to peripheral retinal pathology in the upper half of the posterior segment is difficult when viewed with the operating microscope, and in this situation surgery is best performed using the indirect ophthalmoscope; one port will be required for the cutter, which can be sited in a convenient position.

At the end of any vitrectomy procedure the peripheral retina should be checked with the indirect ophthalmoscope to exclude any incarceration in the sclerotomy sites or oral breaks.

Bacterial Infection

Acute bacterial infection is rare after penetrating eye injuries, except when presentation and treatment have been delayed beyond 24 hours. The flush of aqueous from a penetrating wound helps remove contamination, while the tears have some antibacterial activity.

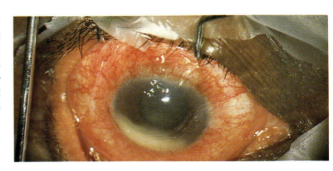

The development of bacterial infection is heralded by increasing pain and deteriorating vision, commencing 24 to 36 hours after injury. Wound infection results in abscess formation with a purulent discharge, and a hypopyon develops in the anterior chamber. Involvement of the posterior segment results in increasing turbidity of the vitreous, with loss of light projection within a few hours.

Fig.7.25 Endophthalmitis with hypopyon and vitreous turbidity.

Management

The initial measures to prevent infection have been described earlier (see page 6.6). If infection develops, a conjunctival smear should be examined to see if any organisms can be recognised, and a wound culture is taken. Appropriate antibiotic therapy is given parenterally together with a daily subconjunctival injection of gentamicin 20 mg and methicillin 150 mg to cover both Gram-negative and Gram-positive organisms. Topical betamethasone and chloramphenicol should be given hourly, plus atropine 1% q.i.d. When the culture report is available, the antibiotic therapy is adjusted according to the sensitivity.

Systemic steroid therapy is commenced after 24 hours of treatment, as this helps counteract the damaging effect of bacterial toxins. Progress should be assessed frequently: if the condition worsens in the next 24 hours, surgical intervention is urgently required. This allows drainage of pus and bacterial toxins, and intraocular fluids can be sampled for further microbiological studies.

Sugery

Visibility is often limited by a corneal abscess or organised exudate in the anterior chamber, and in these cases an anterior approach (see page 7.8) is used; the vitreous cutter is very effective at removing debris and organising material. A pars plana approach (see page 7.9) is preferred when the infection is predominantly affecting the posterior segment. In an aphakic eye this approach still allows access to the anterior segment.

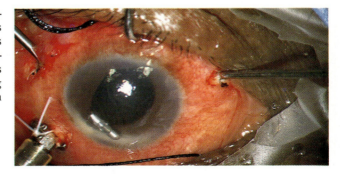

Fig.7.26 Endophthalmitis in an aphakic eye, treated by pars plana vitrectomy.

An intravitreal injection of gentamicin 0.1 mg (intrathecal preparation) plus cephaloridine 0.25 mg is given at the end of surgery. Systemic medication is continued, and in virulent infections further intracameral antibiotic injections should be given after 48 hours.

Effective early treatment can lead to rapid resolution, but if infection has led to abscess formation and widespread intraocular damage, a downhill course ending in evisceration is likely. If the condition stabilises, improvement occurs very slowly over several weeks.

Fungal Infection

This is most likely to occur after an injury due to organic material, and is common after posterior segment trauma because of incomplete removal of contaminants. Symptoms develop after several days, with little pain and a gradual deterioration of vision. A localised grey-white mass forms in the anterior vitreous, which gradually increases or is accompanied by satellite lesions. There may be a transient hypopyon but, in contrast to bacterial infection, light projection is usually well preserved.

In suspected cases, a diagnostic and therapeutic vitrectomy is carried out; smears and cultures are taken as described above, and gentamicin 0.1 mg plus amphotericin B 0.005 mg is injected into the vitreous cavity. Systemic treatment with antifungal agents should be considered when a positive identification of the organism has been made; systemic corticosteroid preparations should not be used.

SYMPATHETIC OPHTHALMITIS

Incidence

Fifty years ago the incidence of this blinding condition after a penetrating eye injury was 20%, and it is still feared today in countries where medical attention is not readily available. With modern treatment, the incidence in this country has fallen to less than 0.5%.

Aetiology

Current research favours an auto-immune process rather than a virus infection, but the exact mechanism is still not fully understood. The stimulus responsible for this condition is thought to be a soluble retinal antigen associated with the photoreceptor and pigment epithelial layer, which is isolated from the immune system in early embryonic development. Similar isolation of lens protein occurs, and both these antigens may be exposed to the immune system after a penetrating injury. Immune-competent cells derived from the conjunctival lymphatic system fail to recognise these antigens as self, and a delayed hypersensitivity reaction develops. Wound contamination may provide an adjuvant effect.

Pathology

The condition is characterised by thickening of the entire uveal tract from widespread infiltration with chronic inflammatory cells; these include sheets of darkly-staining lymphocytes, and paler areas of epithelioid cells, with giant cell formation. These characteristically contain ingested pigment granules.

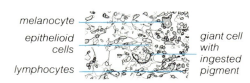

Fig.7.27 Giant cell formation with ingested pigment granules in a patient with sympathetic ophthalmitis. By courtesy of Dr. D.R. Barry.

The epithelioid cells become heaped-up into nodules that protrude into the pigment epithelium (Dalen–Fuchs nodules). These correspond to the disseminated yellow-white spots in the pigment epithelium seen clinically in this condition (see Fig. 7.30).

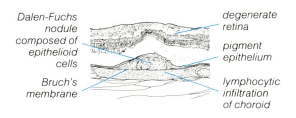

Fig.7.28 Dalen-Fuchs nodule in sympathetic ophthalmitis. By courtesy of Dr. D.R. Barry.

Presentation

The exciting or injured eye remains irritable and initially has a plastic uveitis. Symptoms do not usually develop in the healthy or sympathising eye until four to eight weeks after injury, although they can occur as soon as ten days later or be delayed for over a year. At the onset of sympathetic ophthalmitis, both eyes become increasingly photophobic with a bilateral plastic or granulomatous uveitis, or a profound drop in vision.

The clinical features are similar to the Vogt-Koyanagi-Harada syndrome, and the associated signs of vitiligo, alopecia and poliosis may also occur. The condition is very variable, characterised by remissions and exacerbations, but it never resolves completely.

Anterior involvement

Classically, the initial reactive uveitis in the exciting eye alters, and both eyes develop signs of a chronic granulomatous inflammation. Mild ciliary injection is present, and an aqueous flare with hypotony develops. Characteristically, large mutton–fat keratic precipitates appear on the corneal endothelium.

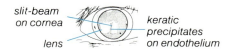

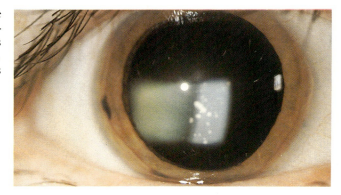

Fig.7.29 Mutton-fat keratic precipitates in sympathetic ophthalmitis.

Posterior involvement

The anterior segment changes can be mild, but a profound reduction in vision occurs from posterior segment involvement; the changes range from macular oedema associated with disseminated small yellow–white spots affecting the pigment epithelium, to more extensive involvement with an exudative retinal detachment.

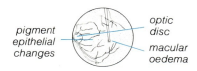

Fig.7.30 Posterior pole oedema and pigment epithelial changes in sympathetic ophthalmitis (see histology of the injured eye, Fig. 7.27).

The fundus appearance is very similar in the Vogt-Koyanagi-Harada syndrome, although in this condition the posterior segment involvement is often more severe, and neurological symptoms are also present.

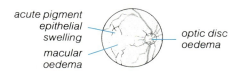

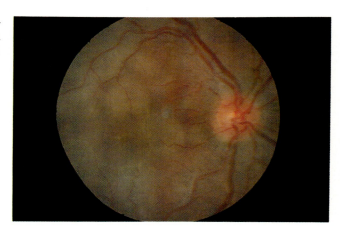

Fig.7.31 Widespread pigment epithelial changes and exudative detachment in Vogt-Koyanagi-Harada syndrome.

Prevention and treatment

Avoidance of tissue incarceration in the wound is important in preventing continued postoperative uveitis, which may predispose to sympathetic ophthalmitis. Since there is a time interval before which the condition is not seen, the policy of enucleating injured eyes damaged beyond repair within ten days of injury helps reduce the incidence of this condition. However, patients with severely injured eyes may not be particularly at risk. The two cases of sympathetic ophthalmitis at our hospital in the last decade both had good acuity in the immediate period after repair. Children have a reactive immunological system, and may be more at risk than adults.

Once the condition is established, the exciting eye should not be excised, as this may ultimately have better vision than the sympathising eye. Local treatment is with 1% atropine q.i.d. and dexamethasone drops hourly, but the mainstay of treatment is systemic steroids (possibly with cytotoxic therapy); very large doses are used initially to control the condition, reducing to a maintenance level when the condition has improved. Long-term treatment is required, which is increased to cover any exacerbations or the stimulus of surgical trauma.

Secondary cataract formation and iris bombé are common complications which may accompany phakoanaphylaxis. Progressive cataract and severe anterior uveitis with cyclitic membrane formation should be tackled surgically, as these can be the main reasons for poor vision; the technique is described on page 8.11.

8

The Management of Anterior Segment Complications

Wound astigmatism

A well-repaired linear corneal laceration should heal with minimal scarring and astigmatism. The refractive error is monitored after repair, and will often show considerable change during the first eight weeks; adjustment of sutures towards the end of this period can help reduce any astigmatic error. If interrupted sutures have been placed at intervals not exceeding 1.5 mm, individual sutures which are too tight can be removed without impairing wound security.

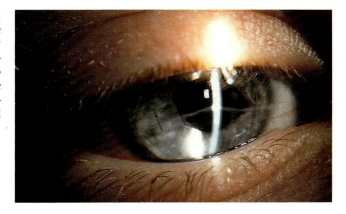

Fig. 8.1 A well-repaired linear wound with minimal scarring and astigmatism: the axial sutures have been removed and a contact lens has been fitted for aphakia.

A laceration complicated by persisting tissue incarceration will result in a vascularised scar with marked astigmatism: the risk is greater with a laceration involving the limbus accompanied by iris, ciliary body and lens damage. Fresh bleeding occurring during repair often obscures the pathology, and early secondary surgery is indicated if the iris or lens capsule remains incarcerated in the wound. If left untreated, irregular scarring and high astigmatism can result, often not amenable to correction.

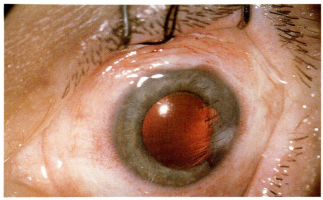

Fig. 8.2 Irregular stress lines from fibrosis of a limbal wound seen against the red reflex during cataract surgery.

Treatment of astigmatism

Regular astigmatism without axial scarring can be corrected with a haptic contact lens, but this may not be tolerated for errors exceeding six dioptres. The surgical options include corneal grafting for central scarring, or relaxing incisions, wedge resections or additional compression sutures for peripheral scarring. If available, an operating keratometer (Terry) is used during these procedures.

Relaxing incisions are used to flatten a steep meridian. 30° deep but non-penetrating incisions are made in the corneal periphery at both ends of the axis of the hypermetropic astigmatism. The cornea is protected with a bandage soft contact lens, and antibiotic drops are instilled regularly until the defect has epithelialised. About four dioptres of astigmatism can be corrected by this method; if necessary, a wedge resection or compression sutures can be performed in the opposite axis to augment the effect.

Wedge resections or compression sutures are used to steepen a flat meridian: the former involves excising a crescentic wedge at one end of the myopic axis, and coapting the edges with interrupted nylon sutures after a paracentesis; the result is not always predictable or easily reversed, and compression sutures are preferred. The aim is to overcorrect the astigmatism, so that selective suture removal can subsequently be carried out to achieve the optimum result.

Compression sutures are placed around the limbus at one or both ends of the more myopic axis; sufficient tension can be achieved with 0.3 metric (9/0) nylon without a paracentesis, if the first triple throw is held prior to completing the knot. Four sutures are placed at two-thirds of depth with 2-3 mm bites and tied tightly to show stress lines in the cornea; the knots are buried by rotation. A 10-15 dioptre change in astigmatism is the immediate result, but it reduces over four to six weeks; persisting overcorrection can be countered by removing individual sutures later. This can be very effective, as the sutures remain intact for a long time.

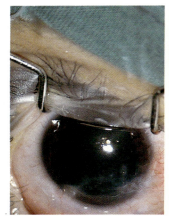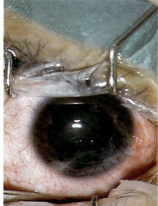

Fig. 8.3 Astigmatism following penetrating trauma improved by compression sutures at the limbus.

Endothelial damage

This results from mechanical damage during the injury and is more likely with shelving corneal lacerations, particularly if foreign material remains within the eye.

During repair, early restoration of the anterior chamber with sodium hyaluronate helps prevent further damage.

Any surgical procedure to the anterior segment results in some loss of endothelial cells, and the risk of decompensation increases with multiple procedures. Before embarking on elective surgery such as secondary implantation of an intraocular lens, endothelial studies should be performed with the specular photomicroscope; if the count falls below the critical level of 1,000 cells per square millimetre, decompensation can occur.

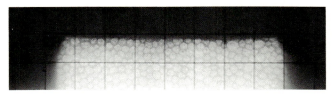

Fig.8.4 Enlarged endothelial cells with a low count seen after an anterior segment perforation (upper), compared to the normal appearance of the uninjured eye (lower).

Penetrating keratoplasty

Keratoplasty may need to be considered for irregular astigmatism, endothelial decompensation or corneal opacification; surgery should either be carried out soon after injury or deferred for at least a year to allow the chronic healing processes to subside.

Stellate wounds affecting the centre of the cornea are the most suitable for corneal grafting. This type of injury is often associated with lens damage, and keratoplasty combined with cataract removal one or two weeks after injury gives the best results. If conditions are favourable, an intraocular lens can be inserted.

Later reconstruction can also be successful for this type of injury; surgery requires cutting of adhesions from the wound after trephining the host cornea, and identifying and cutting capsule remnants if the pupil is occluded. It may be possible to reconstitute the pupil with a 0.2 metric (10/0) polypropylene suture, and secure an iris-supported posterior chamber lens. The keratoplasty is then completed, protecting the endothelium with sodium hyaluronate during suturing.

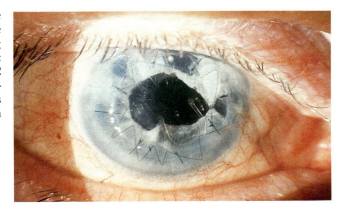

Fig. 8.5 Penetrating keratoplasty for axial scarring, and pupil reconstruction to secure a posterior chamber implant for traumatic aphakia.

An opaque, heavily vascularised cornea is unfavourable for corneal grafting as the risks of rejection are high. This is common after extensive ocular burns, and the associated reduction of tear secretion increases the risk of vascular invasion of the graft, favouring rejection; surgery is best avoided in this situation. However, if the injury affects both eyes, surgery must be considered.

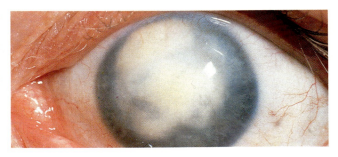

Fig.8.6 An opaque vascularised cornea unfavourable for corneal grafting.

The technique has been described earlier (see page 4.11); it is important to use fresh, young donor material with an intact corneal epithelium. Tissue matching should be carried out prior to surgery. Donor material can be obtained through the UK Transplant Scheme or similar Eye Bank.

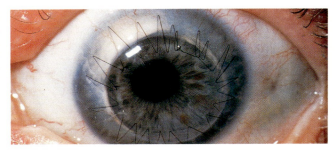

Fig.8.7 Penetrating graft for the above patient. By courtesy of Mr. T.A. Casey.

Lamellar keratoplasty

In some injuries, an axial opacity involves only the superficial layers of the cornea. If the endothelium has not been damaged, lamellar keratoplasty is the treatment of choice, particularly if vascularisation is present. The opacity may not always be due to the injury, but may result from the treatment; a superficial opacity affecting the corneal axis can occur after prolonged wear of a poorly fitting haptic lens for traumatic aphakia.

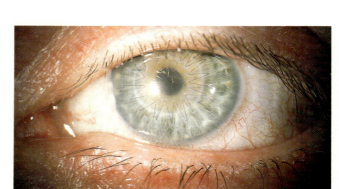

Fig. 8.8 A superficial vascularised opacity after prolonged wear of a poorly fitting contact lens.

If the opacity is small, a rotation keratoplasty can be carried out retaining the patient's own cornea; a larger opacity will require donor material. The best optical results are obtained by a lamellar dissection down to Descemet's membrane. This technique can also be used for a preliminary tectonic graft to build up the thickness and regularity of the cornea prior to a smaller penetrating graft or keratoprosthesis.

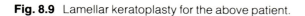

Fig. 8.9 Lamellar keratoplasty for the above patient.

Keratoprosthesis

This procedure is required for desperate situations in patients who are unsuitable for corneal grafting and would otherwise be blind. The prosthesis has a carrying haptic and a central optical portion which needs to project onto both surfaces of the cornea to prevent overgrowth of epithelium and endothelium respectively.

Surgery is carried out in several stages at two to three month intervals: a preliminary tectonic graft may be required to build up the corneal thickness, and lens extraction with division of synechiae is required if the patient is not aphakic.

For a single-piece prosthesis, a deep lamellar split of the whole cornea is performed for the carrying haptic, followed by a full-thickness trephine for the central optical portion. After insertion, the lamellar flap is secured.

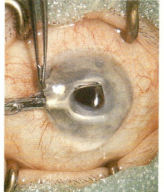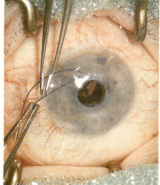

Fig. 8.10 Insertion of a single-piece keratoprosthesis.

In two-piece prostheses, the optical cylinder has a screw fitting so that it can be removed if required. A temporary posterior optic is inserted at the first procedure, leaving the superficial cornea intact. After an interval, the central portion is trephined for insertion of the permanent projecting optic.

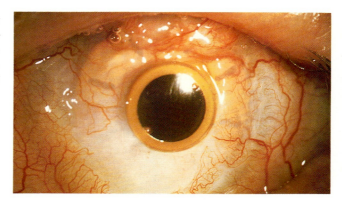

Fig. 8.11 A two-piece Choyce keratoprosthesis.

The two-piece prosthesis has the advantage that the optic can be changed, allowing alteration of the power of the cylinder and division of membranes if these develop on the posterior surface. In the single-piece prosthesis, this complication requires a needling technique.

Glaucoma can arise from anterior synechiae or angle damage from the original injury. It is difficult to assess, because applanation tonometry is impossible and the peripheral visual field is limited by the prosthesis. Digital tension, central visual field analysis and the appearance of the optic disc are monitored, and if medical treatment fails to control the raised pressure, drainage surgery is required (see filtration bleb in Fig. 8.11).

The major problem with keratoprostheses is erosion followed by extrusion, and early tectonic grafting is required if this develops. In this situation, buccal mucous membrane may be more successful than donor cornea.

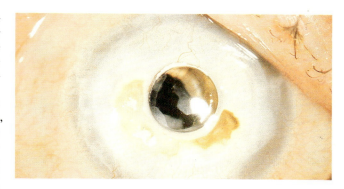

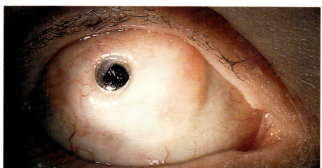

Fig.8.12 A single-piece keratoprosthesis showing erosion six years after insertion (upper); tectonic grafting with buccal mucous membrane allowed successful retention for a further six years (lower).

The Management of Traumatic Cataract

The timing of surgery

There are many factors which influence the timing and method of secondary cataract surgery. In penetrating trauma, when the lens is definitely ruptured, surgical treatment should be carried out at primary repair. When there is doubt about this, or lens damage results from a blunt injury or the passage of a small intraocular foreign body, surgery is deferred until evidence of progressive opacification occurs.

The cataract should be removed before it becomes swollen as this increases the risk of complications from lens rupture, uveitis and glaucoma and makes the surgery more difficult.

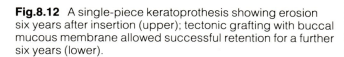

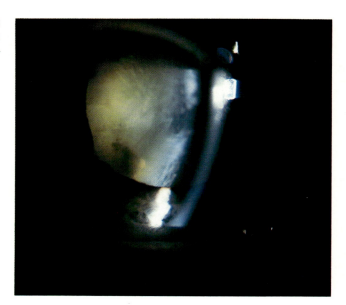

Fig. 8.13 Shallowing of the anterior chamber due to an intumescent cataract with an intralenticular foreign body.

The sudden development of uveitis and rapid progression of cataract with an intact anterior capsule should suggest a posterior lens rupture, which can be confirmed by the ultrasonographic appearance (see page 7.3). In this case urgent surgical intervention is required.

Concussion injuries with progressive cataract often have associated macular damage (see page 5.12). In the absence of uveitis or lens swelling, surgery should be deferred for six months if possible, to allow recovery from macular oedema.

In injuries accompanied by posterior segment haemorrhage, early surgery may precipitate fresh bleeding; unless the lens is ruptured, lens surgery is deferred for four to six weeks. Vitrectomy may also be required, and combined lens and vitreous surgery is then carried out through a pars plana approach.

8.5

Lens aspiration or lensectomy

In most cases, the traumatic cataract has followed a penetrating injury, and the patient is usually young; lens aspiration or lensectomy is indicated. The pupil is dilated prior to surgery with 1% cyclopentolate and 1% atropine drops; this is maintained during surgery by an infusion of balanced salt solution containing 1 in 100,000 adrenaline.

The surgical approach is similar for either primary or secondary lens removal: in the former, wound toilet and closure are performed first. The damaged lens is removed as a closed procedure through two 20-gauge corneal or limbal incisions. If the anterior capsule is intact, a preliminary anterior capsulotomy is performed with an irrigating capsulotomy needle.

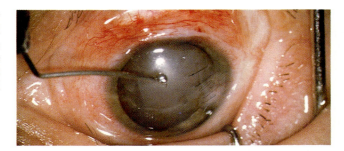

Fig. 8.14 An irrigating needle for anterior capsulotomy.

In many traumatic cataracts, liquefaction and swelling of the lens has occurred and removal of the anterior capsule can be difficult. In this situation an anterior capsulotomy using saline irrigation is followed by immediate prolapse of soft lens matter into the anterior chamber, often followed by the nucleus. This causes a linear split of the anterior capsule, leaving large flaps which interfere with subsequent lens removal.

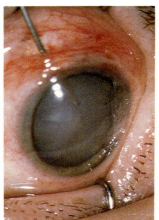
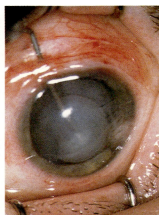

Fig. 8.15 Anterior capsulotomy (left), followed by forward dislocation of the nucleus in a swollen traumatic cataract (right).

This sudden rupture of the lens can be prevented by filling the anterior chamber with sodium hyaluronate prior to performing the capsulotomy. This allows a controlled anterior capsulotomy to be performed. In this way, complete removal of the anterior capsule can be achieved without resorting to other cutting instruments.

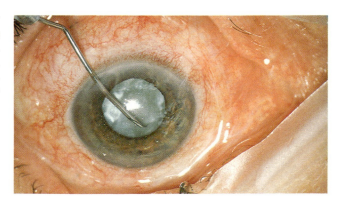

Fig. 8.16 Anterior capsulotomy in a swollen cataract using sodium hyaluronate to prevent splitting of the anterior capsule.

After removing the anterior capsule, the lens matter can be easily removed. A simple infusion-aspiration device can be used if the posterior capsule is intact, but if there is doubt about this, a vitreous cutter is preferred. Variable suction that can be operated through a foot control gives greater safety and leaves both hands free for instrumentation.

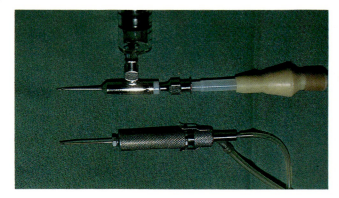

Fig. 8.17 A disposable lens-aspiration needle compared to a vitreous cutter.

A bimanual technique, using the cutter in one hand and a blunt 20-gauge needle connected to an infusion line in the other, is preferable to using a single incision and an infusion sleeve; the former gives greater control and allows exchange of instruments to reach difficult areas. Soft lens matter is aspirated first, followed by removal of any remaining flaps of anterior capsule using either intraocular scissors or the vitreous cutter; the nucleus can then be aspirated.

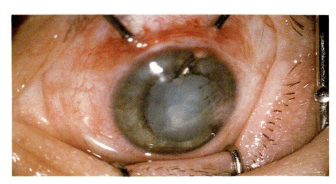

Fig. 8.18 Bimanual technique during lens removal.

Suction is used to peel the remaining lens cortex from the periphery towards the centre, where it can be removed by increased suction alternating with the cutting mode. All cortical lens matter should be removed, and in children under seven years a wide posterior capsulotomy should always be performed. The incisions are then closed with 0.2 metric (10/0) nylon and the knots buried.

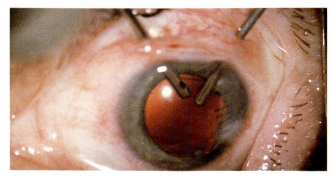

Fig. 8.19 Lens removal nearing completion.

If the posterior capsule is defective, vitreous will prolapse into the anterior chamber during surgery, and effective aspiration becomes impossible. The vitreous cutter is essential in this situation for dealing with the lens/vitreous mixture. Wide removal of the posterior capsule should be performed at the completion of surgery.

If the posterior capsule is left intact after lens aspiration or extracapsular extraction (see below),

thickening is likely to occur after an interval of time, especially in the younger age group. This can be countered by a small posterior capsulotomy performed at the end of surgery after injecting sodium hyaluronate. If this is not performed, or the gap subsequently closes, secondary capsulotomy is often required. Yag laser techniques have recently been developed which allow this to be performed as an outpatient procedure.

Extracapsular removal

In the older age group the nucleus will be too dense for aspiration, requiring either phako-emulsification or a larger section for removal. In the latter the wound is enlarged after the anterior capsule has been removed, and the nucleus is expressed or removed with a vectis after filling the anterior chamber with sodium hyaluronate. The section is then closed before proceeding.

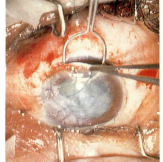 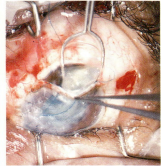

Fig. 8.20 Extracapsular extraction of the nucleus in a traumatic cataract.

Intracapsular removal

An intracapsular extraction can be performed, which is often a safer approach after the passage of a small intraocular foreign body; a defect in the posterior capsule can give way during extracapsular surgery, which can result in posterior displacement of the nucleus.

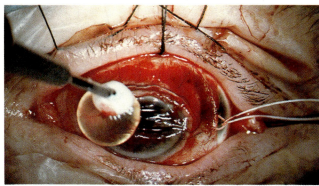

Fig. 8.21 Intracapsular cataract extraction after exploring a posterior segment foreign body (double perforation).

8.7

The Management of Posterior Lens Displacements

Major lens displacements are obvious and usually result from severe concussion injuries; hyphaema and extensive angle damage are common, and the vitreous is displaced and often haemorrhagic. A similar lens displacement can complicate an anterior scleral rupture.

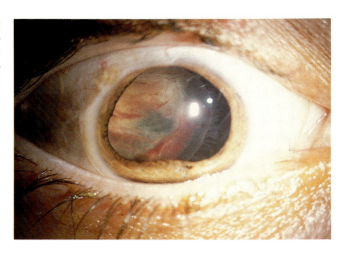

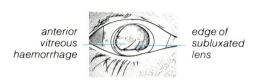

Fig.8.22 A subluxated lens and vitreous haemorrhage after a scleral rupture.

Minor lens displacements are less obvious, but should be suspected in any cataract occurring after blunt injury; iridodonesis (trembling of the iris diaphragm on eye movement) should suggest this, while maximal pupil dilation often reveals the zonular defect.

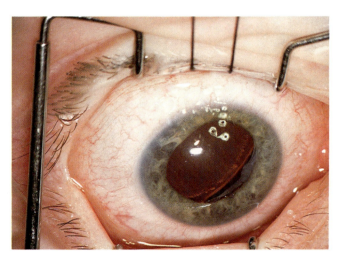

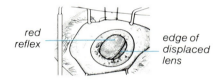

Fig.8.23 Mild lens subluxation revealed on full pupil dilation.

An extensive rupture of the zonule can result in a posteriorly dislocated lens which hinges about a point of residual attachment; this can interfere with vision because the lens position varies with posture. A complete posterior lens dislocation usually settles in the inferior vitreous, but if the latter is degenerate, the lens can remain mobile.

Surgery is indicated if the vision deteriorates because of progressive cataract, or if displacement of a clear lens interferes with vision either from high astigmatism because the edge of the lens is lying in the visual axis, or because of changes of lens position with posture. A complete posterior dislocation can be left alone if stable, unless uveitis, vitreous reaction and glaucoma supervene.

Removal of a Posterior Subluxated Lens

Subluxated lenses are unsuitable for extracapsular cataract extraction as vitreous will often prolapse into the anterior chamber during surgery; the choice is between intracapsular extraction or lensectomy.

The former approach is used for removal of an extensively dislocated lens hinged about a residual zonular attachment or, in the older age group, with a dense nucleus. If significantly displaced, the lens will first require stabilising with a large-radius needle introduced through the pars plana behind the point of hinging. The tip should be directed posteriorly to engage the opposite pole of the lens which can then be manoeuvred forwards; removal is then carried out through a standard cataract section. The needle site should be examined at the end of the procedure to check that no vitreous has been drawn into the wound. This procedure carries the risk of posterior segment damage from vitreous base traction or direct retinal damage if the needle is inserted too posteriorly.

Closed removal using a vitreous cutter is preferable in young patients with incomplete traumatic dislocations where the remaining vitreo-lenticular attachments are strong; an intracapsular extraction can lead to traction on the vitreous base and retinal complications. With significant subluxation a pars plana approach is needed to obtain access to the displaced lens. This approach is also needed for lens displacement complicating an anterior scleral rupture with vitreous haemorrhage, as vitrectomy will also be required.

8.8

The procedure is carried out through the pars plana and a separate infusion line is sutured in position (see page 7.9). A preliminary anterior vitrectomy is performed to allow adequate infusion.

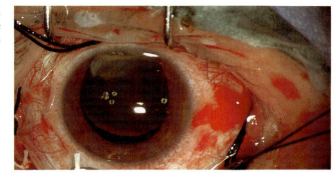

Fig. 8.24 A subluxated lens complicating an anterior scleral laceration: an infusion line has been inserted and preliminary anterior vitrectomy performed.

The lens capsule is then penetrated by the sclerotomy blade or needle via the standard pars plana incision, and the vitreous probe is introduced into the lens for controlled removal of the cortex and nucleus from within the capsule. The procedure is viewed through the illuminated microscope, but additional retro–illumination with the fibreoptic probe helps identify the structures.

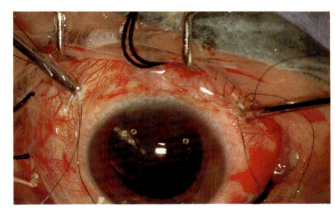

Fig.8.25 Preliminary needle puncture of the lens.

If available, phako–emulsification of the lens speeds up the removal, but if not available, the suction and cutting modes are used alternately to aspirate the lens. Initially a fairly high level of suction is required, and the cortex can be peeled away from the capsule in the usual way.

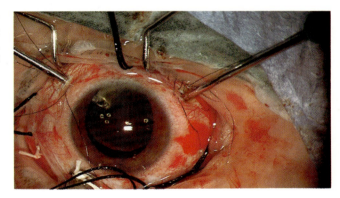

Fig. 8.26 Removing the lens material within the capsular bag.

After removing the lens material, the posterior capsule is excised with the cutter, but the anterior capsule is left until the end of the procedure, to protect the corneal endothelium from the infusion. The posterior segment is examined with the contact lens in position to check for any lens fragments, and the peripheral retina is examined with the indirect ophthalmoscope after temporary closure of the ports. After completing any vitreous surgery, the anterior capsule is removed with the vitreous cutter prior to closure.

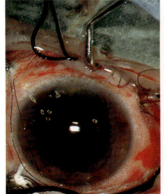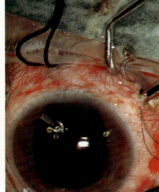

Fig. 8.27 Appearance before and after excising the anterior capsule.

A pars plana approach is also used for long-standing total posterior lens dislocations that require removal because of complications. A preliminary vitrectomy is performed to expose the cataractous lens; during this procedure the capsule often ruptures and must be removed with any soft lens matter using the cutter. The nucleus is too hard for removal, and care must be taken not to push it against the retina causing damage. It is lifted and supported by strong suction until it is brought up to the anterior chamber; the pupil is then constricted behind the nucleus with acetylcholine via the infusion line, and after closing the ports, it is removed via a limbal section using sodium hyaluronate to protect the endothelium.

8.9

The Management of Anterior Lens Displacements

This usually causes pupil block and a rapid rise of intraocular pressure. The patient presents with an acute red eye, with severe supraorbital pain, vomiting and prostration. The cornea is hazy from raised intraocular pressure, but the outline of the clear lens can be seen in the anterior chamber.

The medical treatment has been discussed on page 5.10. If this fails to bring down the intraocular pressure with an anterior dislocation, emergency surgery to the lens is necessary. Preoperatively, mannitol 1.5g/kg is given intravenously to help reduce the intraocular pressure; general anaesthetic techniques can also reduce the vascular congestion and vitreous volume prior to opening the eye. A controlled release of aqueous via a needle-puncture makes the subsequent procedure much softer.

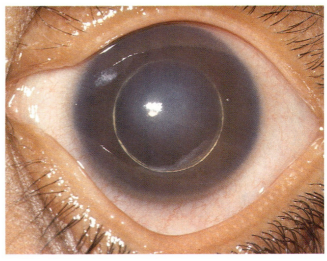

Fig. 8.28 A clear lens dislocated into the anterior chamber.

A peripheral iridectomy is performed first to overcome the pupil block. The pupil is then constricted behind the lens using acetylcholine, and sodium hyaluronate is injected into the anterior chamber. Closed microsurgical removal of the lens is carried out through two small corneal incisions, using an infusion needle and vitreous cutter as described earlier. This approach is safer than attempting intracapsular extraction in an eye that has been under considerable pressure, where there is a significant risk of an expulsive haemorrhage. If medical treatment overcomes the pupil block and the dislocated lens returns to the posterior chamber, a peripheral iridectomy is required to prevent further attacks. Laser techniques can be used for this.

A peripheral iridectomy is also used in the early management of forward subluxation of the lens behind the iris, causing pupil block and an acute rise of intraocular pressure (see Fig. 5.15). Later cataract formation generally occurs and an intracapsular extraction is then the procedure of choice.

Late Management of Traumatic Cataract

In some patients, the traumatic cataract is slow in developing, and insertion of an intraocular lens at the time of cataract removal can be considered. There are some absolute contraindications such as an unhealthy endothelium or extensive angle recession with raised intraocular pressure. Damage to the posterior segment is a relative contraindication, but lens implantation can be considered if it has been possible to assess and monitor any minor posterior segment damage.

The nature of the original injury and type of damage will often determine the surgical procedure and design of implant. As discussed earlier, traumatic cataract complicating blunt injury often has a weakened zonule making extracapsular extraction unsuitable. Similarly cataracts that develop after the passage of a small intraocular foreign body have a weakened posterior capsule, and intracapsular surgery is the safest approach. The type of lens implant will depend on pupil function and the integrity or otherwise of the posterior capsule; a posterior chamber lens is preferable (supported by the iris or posterior capsule according to the surgery), but in some cases an anterior chamber implant is the only alternative.

In some cases a damaged lens has been allowed to absorb spontaneously, which may leave a thickened capsular remnant with posterior synechiae. This will need excising, as it is too thick for division with Yag laser. A closed microsurgical approach is the procedure of choice for a cyclitic membrane associated with uveitis (see pages 8.11-12), but in a quiet eye with a stable intraocular pressure an open approach allows pupil reconstruction and lens implantation. Associated corneal damage may require grafting if the axis of vision is involved, but peripheral scarring can be left.

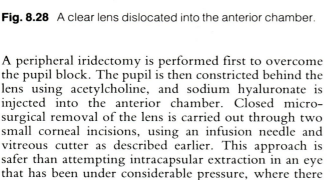

Fig. 8.29 An anterior segment perforation requiring reconstruction.

After a preliminary corneal section, anterior synechiae to the wound can be divided with scissors, and any bleeding can be controlled by using the intraocular bipolar cautery probe. The synechiae between iris and lens are often quite tenuous and are separated with an iris repositor, or injection of sodium hyaluronate.

With shrunken capsule remnants, complete removal is often possible after enzymatic zonulysis, using either capsule forceps or a cryoprobe. Pupil reconstruction is then performed with 0.2 metric (10/0) nylon or polypropylene.

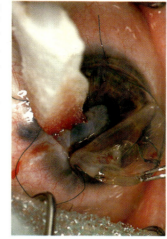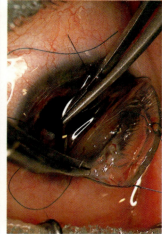

Fig.8.30 left & right Separating posterior synechiae and reconstructing the pupil after removal of lens remnants.

This allows insertion of an iris-supported posterior chamber lens using sodium hyaluronate into the anterior chamber. Good results can be expected if the injury has been confined to the anterior segment.

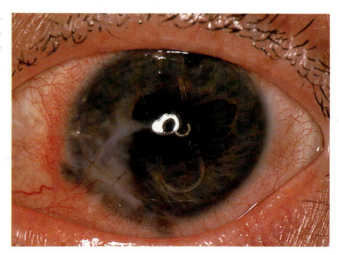

Fig.8.31 Postoperative appearance of the above patient, with 6/9 vision.

The Management of Hypotony from Cyclitic Membrane Formation

An anterior injury that involves both lens rupture and a laceration involving the ciliary body with anterior vitreous haemorrhage will lead to severe anterior segment fibrosis if not treated at an early stage. The inflammatory response in the eye promotes anterior vitreous fibrosis and formation of a cyclitic membrane; this leads to ciliary body detachment and hypotony, and ultimately to retinal detachment.

Clinically these injured eyes have persisting uveitis, low intraocular pressure, and a bound-down pupil with total posterior synechiae and iris bombé. Initially, light projection is preserved (except in cases following infection), and electrodiagnostic tests should confirm good retinal function.

The downhill course can be arrested by radical anterior segment surgery; in a soft eye, an anterior approach via two small limbal incisions is preferred, as the ciliary body may be detached. Infusion is provided via a blunt 20-gauge needle in one hand, while the cutter or other 20-gauge instruments are used in the other. The membrane needs incising first with a capsulotomy knife, which is then segmented with scissors and removed with the vitreous cutter. Synechiae to the wound can be divided with scissors.

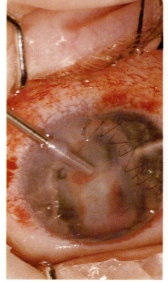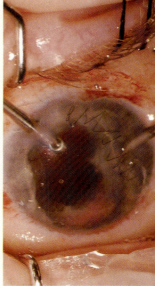

Fig.8.32 left & right An anterior approach to a cyclitic membrane, using the above techniques.

If the intraocular pressure is maintained but iris bombé is present, a pars plana approach is used. A preliminary infusion line is set up (for details see page 7.9) in the lower temporal quadrant 3 mm behind the limbus. The sclerotomy blade is introduced deeply into the vitreous cavity to be certain of penetration, and a 6 mm infusion needle is used. Two similar sclerotomies are made above into the vitreous cavity, and the membrane is incised with a capsulotomy needle prior to preliminary removal of lens remnants (see Fig.5.15).

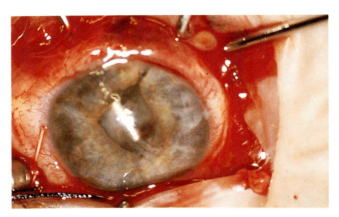

Fig. 8.33 Iris bombé and cyclitic membrane after a dart injury and infection: infusion line prepared and preliminary removal of lens remnants.

It is usually necessary to remove the pupil margin, as this is firmly adherent to the cyclitic membrane. If bleeding occurs at this stage it can be controlled by intraocular bipolar wet-field cautery. The power should be turned down to a low level before testing the probe on iris tissue; coagulation is accompanied by a stream of tiny bubbles of water vapour.

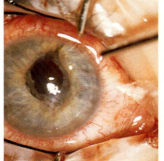 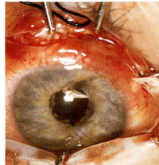

Once the iris is free, a plane between this and the underlying membrane can be identified. Fine angled intraocular scissors are used to make radial cuts in the membrane to reduce the tension on the ciliary body. When the membrane is relaxed and segmented, the vitreous cutter can complete the removal. The iris bombé usually resolves during the procedure, but if not, the anterior chamber can be established with sodium hyaluronate via a paracentesis.

Fig.8.34 left & right Identifying and segmenting the cyclitic membrane.

After removing the cyclitic membrane, the posterior segment is inspected with the fibreoptic light and the contact lens on the cornea. Sometimes fragments of lens fall back into the vitreous cavity, and these should be removed by aspiration. After closure of the ports with 0.3 metric (9/0) nylon, the peripheral retina is inspected with the indirect ophthalmoscope.

Relief of ciliary body traction usually results in a dramatic improvement in the condition of the eye: the uveitis settles and the intraocular pressure recovers, unless hypotony has been present for some time. In this case, extensive choroidal and ciliary body detachment may persist, and the intraocular pressure is slow to recover. The outcome can be disappointing in young children, as aggressive fibroplasia is common, and the membrane may reform.

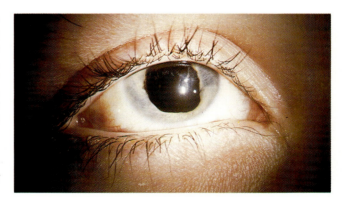

Fig. 8.35 The postoperative appearance of the above injury four weeks after surgery.

The posterior segment must be carefully assessed in the postoperative period. Epiretinal fibrosis is often present preventing the retina flattening as the choroidal effusions absorb, or there may be posterior segment damage related to the previous injury. An encircling procedure is required after a period of recovery to support the vitreous base region.

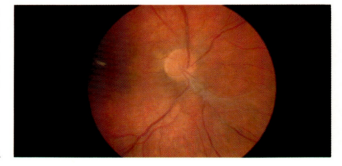

Fig. 8.36 Fundus appearance of the above injury four weeks after surgery, showing residual epiretinal membranes.

The options for unilateral aphakia are contact lens fitting or an intraocular lens. In many patients, lens surgery has been carried out as part of the primary repair for a perforating injury, and if a satisfactory correction can be achieved with a contact lens, this is the safest approach.

Continuous-wear soft haptic lenses are the easiest to fit in children (see Fig. 8.1), but are not without complications; repeated episodes of infection with corneal ulceration can occur, and this may leave corneal opacities and

vascularisation. If sufficiently co-operative, daily wear-soft or hard lenses are fitted, which reduces the risk of infection.

Many young adults fail to continue with contact lens wear because of discomfort, double vision, or the nuisance involved when they have good sight in the other eye. A secondary implant can be considered after an adequate trial of a contact lens, particularly if their occupation demands good vision in both eyes.

Suitable injuries are perforations confined to the anterior segment. If the pupil is atonic after blunt trauma, an iris-supported lens is impracticable, and the choice is between a posterior or anterior chamber lens; the former is preferable, but may not be possible if synechiae between iris and capsule are present, or the posterior capsule is defective.

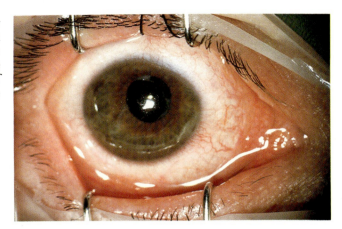

Fig. 8.37 Traumatic aphakia and failed contact lens wear after blunt injury.

The endothelial count should be checked before surgery, and if favourable, the implant is inserted via a small corneal or limbal incision using air or sodium hyaluronate to maintain the anterior chamber. The procedure causes minimal disturbance with immediate improvement in vision. Orthoptic treatment is sometimes required postoperatively if a long-standing divergent squint has been present; occasionally secondary muscle surgery may be required.

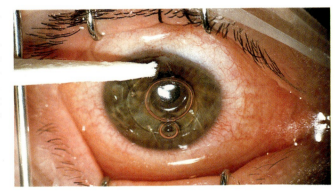

Fig. 8.38 Secondary insertion of an anterior chamber implant.

In bilateral traumatic aphakia, the choice is between spectacles or contact lenses. Before seat-belt legislation, windscreen lacerations often caused bilateral perforations with aphakia and aniridia. Although painted haptic lenses improve both vision and the appearance, tolerance may be limited as these are often compromised corneas. Spectacle correction with plastic aspheric lenses incorporating a suitable tint will often be required.

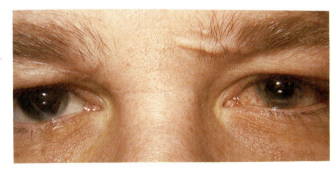

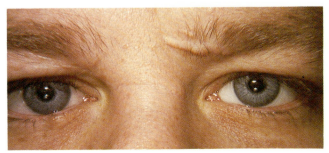

Fig. 8.39 upper & lower Bilateral traumatic aniridia and aphakia, with haptic contact lenses.

If surgery is required for traumatic cataract, iris defects such as a sector iridectomy can be reconstructed using 0.2 metric (10/0) nylon or polypropylene (see page 8.11). In some patients, however, large iris defects occur in the absence of lens damage, and iris reconstruction should be considered for troublesome photophobia.

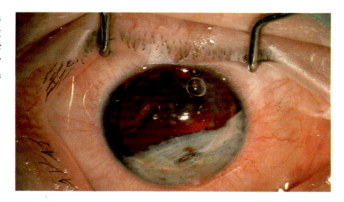

Fig.8.40 A penetrating injury of the cornea complicated by an extensive iridodialysis.

Surgery carries the risk of damaging a clear lens, but the use of sodium hyaluronate has made reconstruction much safer. The anterior chamber is first deepened with sodium hyaluronate via a paracentesis. The iris can then be separated from the lens by injecting sodium hyaluronate between these two structures, using a fine angled canula (Rycroft).

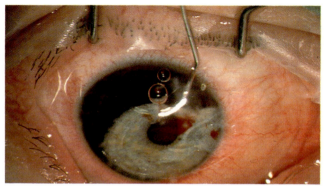

Fig.8.41 Freeing iris synechiae from the lens using sodium hyaluronate.

Once free, the iris limb can be gently mobilised into a better position prior to fixation (if not secured, the iris tissue will fall back into its preoperative position). The initial paracentesis is closed at this stage, so that the eye is watertight before proceeding.

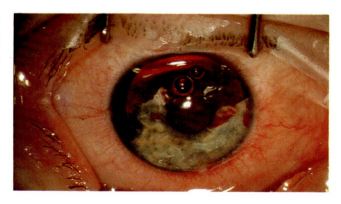

Fig.8.42 The torn iris mobilised into a better anatomical position.

The conjunctiva is reflected away from the limbus at the site chosen for fixation, and a small corneoscleral section is made. Using sodium hyaluronate to maintain the anterior chamber depth, the iris tissue is drawn into the wound using fine forceps, and 0.2 metric (10/0) polypropylene sutures are passed through iris tissue. Loose knots are formed leaving the suture ends attached; the iris is then reposited into the anterior chamber and the wound closed separately with 0.2 metric (10/0) nylon, passing the needle through the polypropylene loops. The latter are trimmed close to the knot before the wound is closed.

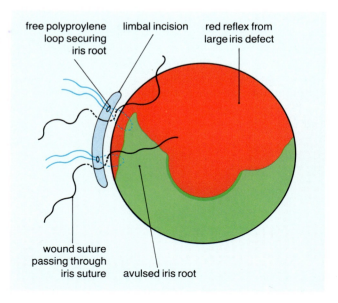

Fig.8.43 Diagram showing method of securing an iridodialysis.

In the early period after injury complications such as hyphaema, lens dislocation and rupture mechanically block aqueous flow leading to an acute rise of pressure, and require urgent treatment as previously described.

Intractable glaucoma can follow a severe blunt injury after an initial period of hypotony. Widespread damage includes extensive angle recession, cyclodialysis, lens subluxation or cataract, and dense vitreous haemorrhage.

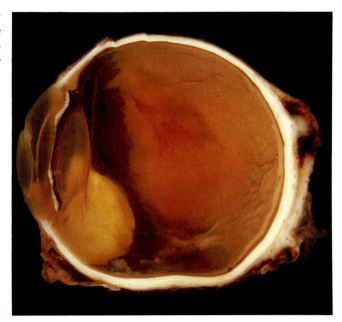

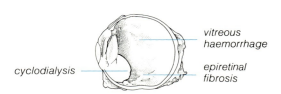

Fig.8.44 An enucleated eye following severe blunt trauma, showing a cyclodialysis and early preretinal fibrosis. By courtesy of Prof. W.R. Lee.

The raised pressure is due to red cell products clogging a compromised outflow pathway, and uveitis associated with lens damage and vitreous haemorrhage. The initial treatment should be conservative (see page 5.11), as surgical intervention is likely to be complicated by further bleeding. Assessment should include serial ultrasonography and electrodiagnostic tests (see pages 7.3-4), and if retinal detachment is suspected, a pars plana vitrectomy and retinal surgery are carried out (see pages 9.12-13); the prognosis is generally poor.

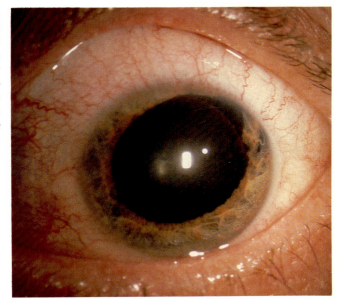

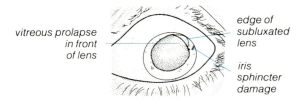

Fig.8.45 Vitreous prolapse in front of lens and damage of the iris sphincter.

If retinal function is normal but uveitis and raised pressure continue with progressive cataract formation, lensectomy plus anterior vitrectomy (see page 8.9) should be considered. A trabeculectomy can be subsequently performed if required. If the intraocular pressure is very high but the eye is quiet without cataract formation, a trabeculectomy is performed initially, but should this fail, a pars plana vitrectomy must be considered.

Late glaucoma

This can develop due to a variety of causes, years after injury. It may occur after extensive angle recession from blunt trauma (see page 5.9), but is also common after extensive perforating injuries with aniridia and aphakia. The element of contusion in these injuries causes angle damage, and protracted uveitis or tissue incarceration in a wound will leave extensive anterior synechiae which mechanically obstruct the angle. All these factors may impair aqueous outflow and eventually lead to glaucoma: regular assessment of patients at risk is required. In complicated injuries, medical therapy is the treatment of choice.

Epithelialisation of the anterior chamber

An uncommon cause of raised intraocular pressure is epithelialisation of the anterior chamber; this can occur if an injury is neglected and repair delayed. Sheets of epithelium grow over the iris, angle and posterior corneal surface, and ultimately spread posteriorly over the ciliary body and anterior vitreous.

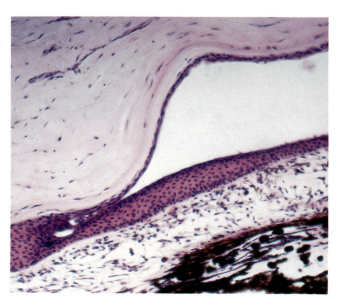

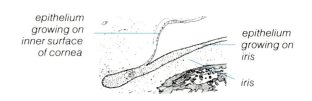

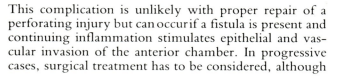

Fig.8.46 Histological appearance of epithelialisation of the anterior chamber. By courtesy of Dr. J. Harry.

This complication is unlikely with proper repair of a perforating injury but can occur if a fistula is present and continuing inflammation stimulates epithelial and vascular invasion of the anterior chamber. In progressive cases, surgical treatment has to be considered, although the outlook is poor; treatment consists of closing the fistula and excising the accessible epithelial tissue, followed by cryotherapy to areas not accessible to removal.

9

The Management of Posterior Segment Complications

Vitreous haemorrhage after a closed eye injury is not associated with the risk of intraocular fibrosis that occurs with a penetrating wound, and conservative management is usually adopted. The commonest indication for pars plana vitrectomy after blunt ocular trauma is vitreous haemorrhage associated with a giant retinal tear (see page 9.13). Rarely, intractable glaucoma associated with a dense vitreous haemorrhage is an indication for vitrectomy, as discussed on page 8.15.

An infusion line and entry ports for the vitreous cutter and fibreoptic light are prepared as described earlier (page 7.9). The procedure is carried out with a contact lens that allows focusing on the posterior structures. Internal illumination by the fibreoptic light pipe gives the best visibility, keeping the tip slightly behind the cutter to avoid reflections. The instruments are introduced with the microscope illuminated, but once visible behind the lens, the microscope light is extinguished, leaving the focus and zoom mechanisms operational. All foot controls should be within reach and operated smoothly.

Visibility is often limited initially, and experience is required to judge the position of the instruments. A glimmer of light from the fibreoptic probe and movement of the anterior gel can be seen as the cutter is used to obtain clearance behind the lens.

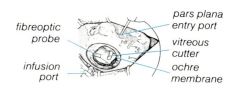

Fig.9.1 The cutter and fibreoptic probe in the anterior vitreous before positioning the contact lens.

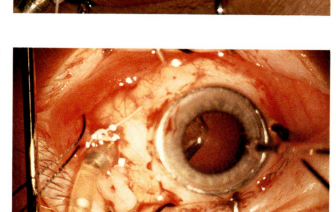

After positioning the contact lens on the cornea, the microscope is focused down as the instruments are moved more posteriorly. The contact lens reduces the size of the image, so the zoom facility is used to increase the magnification. The bimanual technique allows the globe to be rotated in different directions to reach less accessible parts.

Fig.9.2 The irrigating contact lens in position.

The aim is to clear a path through the detached posterior vitreous face, keeping away from any point of fixed attachment such as the optic disc. Once a gap is obtained the retina can be inspected and its relation to the remaining vitreous established.

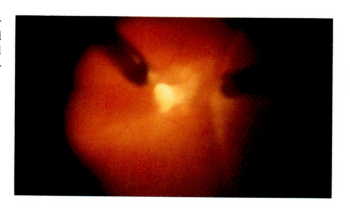

Fig.9.3 Detached retina illuminated by the fibreoptic light viewed through a gap in the ochre membrane.

When working near the retina the cutting aperture and suction pressure are reduced while the cutting rate is increased to reduce any vitreous traction on the retina. This is particularly important if the retina is detached.

After completing the vitrectomy, the entry ports are closed (see page 7.9) and the retina is examined with the indirect ophthalmoscope; any retinal breaks will require treatment, as discussed later (page 9.13).

Vitreous haemorrhage combined with a penetrating wound is a potent stimulus to fibroplasia (see discussion on page 7.6). In transected globes, expulsion of intraocular contents including the lens and most of the vitreous leaves little scaffold for fibrosis, and although posterior segment haemorrhage is often present, vitrectomy is rarely required.

Injuries resulting in smaller posterior wounds, without major vitreous loss but with diffuse vitreous haemorrhage, are most at risk in developing the complications of intraocular fibrosis. This is likely to complicate scleral lacerations or injuries from large intraocular foreign bodies.

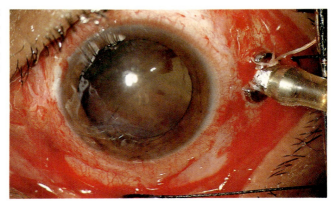

Fig.9.4 Diffuse vitreous haemorrhage after removal of a posterior segment intraocular foreign body.

In scleral lacerations, the fibrosis originates anteriorly from the wound and extends tangentially in the vitreous base. If dense vitreous haemorrhage is not removed surgically, the subsequent fibrosis leads to progressive traction on the adjacent vitreous base, retina and lens, with ultimate displacement. Vitrectomy should be carried out before these changes develop.

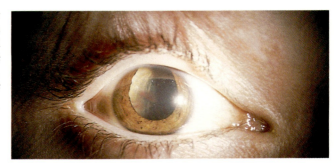

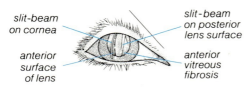

slit-beam on cornea
slit-beam on posterior lens surface
anterior surface of lens
anterior vitreous fibrosis

Fig.9.5 upper & lower Anterior vitreous fibrosis four months after a superior scleral laceration and vitreous haemorrhage.

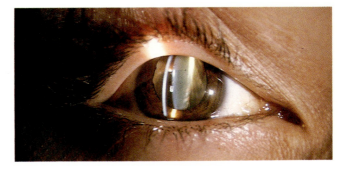

Intraocular foreign bodies with dense vitreous haemorrhage have invariably sustained damage to the posterior retina; this together with the entry wound or extraction site provide multiple sources for fibroplasia. If the stimulus to fibrosis is not removed, anteroposterior traction develops.

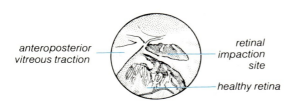

anteroposterior vitreous traction
retinal impaction site
healthy retina

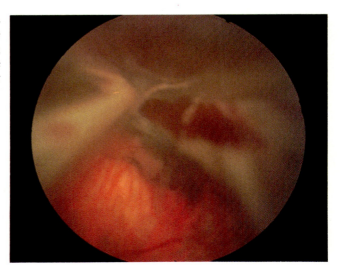

Fig.9.6 Anteroposterior traction following removal of an intraocular foreign body from the posterior segment.

Although the posterior scar resists the traction for a long period, progressive elevation may occur accompanied by subretinal exudate and fibrosis; rhegmatogenous retinal detachment can also occur from traction on the vitreous base resulting in a small oral break.

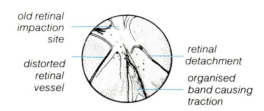
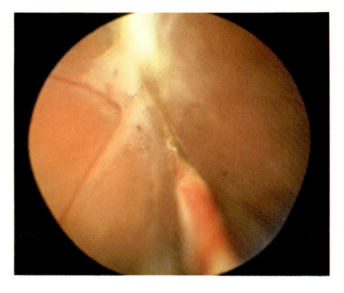

old retinal impaction site

distorted retinal vessel

retinal detachment

organised band causing traction

Fig.9.7 Transgel traction from an intraocular foreign body causing localised posterior retinal detachment.

Surgery

Vitrectomy can be undertaken a week after injury when the posterior vitreous has separated from the retina. However, most injuries have resulted in significant contusion, and early surgery has a high risk of secondary bleeding. To avoid this, vitrectomy is usually carried out between two to six weeks after injury. Preoperative assessment (see pages 7.2–4) with ultrasonography and electrodiagnostic tests is important to help determine the extent of posterior segment damage.

The majority of these injuries will have some fibrosis affecting the vitreous base, and an encircling procedure is required. This is usually sutured in position at the start of surgery, but not tightened until completion of the vitrectomy.

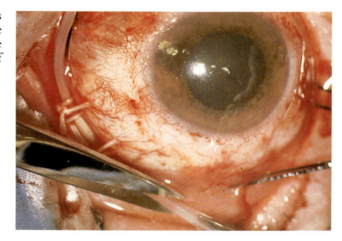

Fig.9.8 An encircling band prepared prior to vitrectomy.

If there is an anterior scleral wound, the ports should be made as far away from it as possible, in case a localised retinal separation is already present; if fibrosis of the vitreous base is already established, the organised tissue resists the passage of the sclerotomy blade and produces a retinal dialysis. The safest approach is to perform the vitrectomy through a single cutting port sited well away from the wound, using the indirect ophthalmoscope.

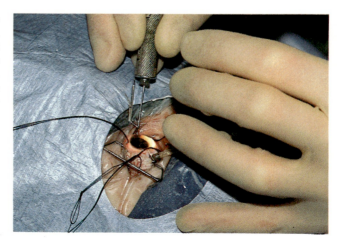

Fig.9.9 Preparing for vitrectomy using the indirect ophthalmoscope.

A clear lens should be preserved where possible, and to avoid damage, the cutting port should be located posteriorly (4.0 mm behind the limbus), as the probe will need to cross the globe obliquely. If the lens is damaged or involved in organised tissue, a preliminary lensectomy is performed (see page 8.8).

Vitrectomy following an intraocular foreign body is more straightforward, as the pathology is predominantly posterior and accessible using the operating microscope.

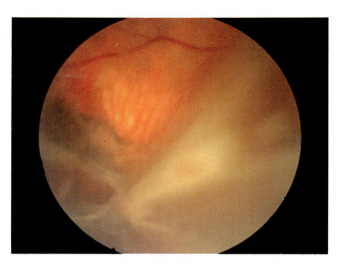

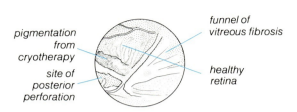

Fig.9.10 Vitreous fibrosis to a posterior retinal scar following double perforation by an intraocular foreign body.

If surgery is delayed, the organised tissue becomes quite taut, and requires cutting with intraocular scissors; once released, the vitreous cutter can amputate the stumps.

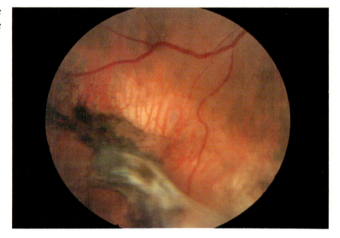

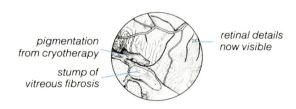

Fig.9.11 Postoperative appearance after vitrectomy and encirclement in the same patient.

The outcome following early vitrectomy for anterior scleral lacerations is often good as the posterior pole has escaped damage. After an intraocular foreign body, the visual outcome can be marred by damage to the macular region. Localised epiretinal fibrosis is common, causing distortion of the structures at the posterior pole.

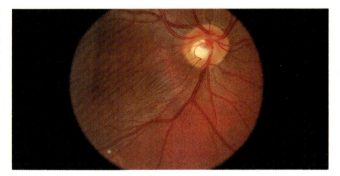

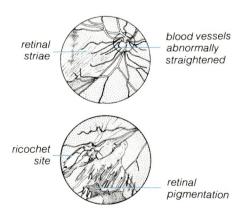

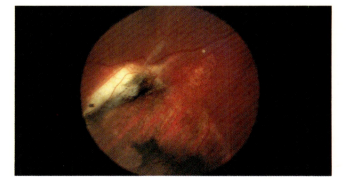

Fig.9.12 upper & lower Macular drag from a posterior ricochet site of a foreign body.

The incidence of retinal detachment after posterior segment perforations has fallen from 20% to about 5% following the introduction of vitrectomy techniques; in some patients severe epiretinal fibrosis rapidly develops, leading to a disappointing outcome. Other reasons for failure include retinal incarceration, or delayed surgery allowing fibrosis and traction detachment to develop; complications are likely to be higher in this group.

9.5

Posterior foreign bodies without vitreous haemorrhage

Small steel particles located posteriorly can be beyond the range of the electromagnet, and if extraction fails by this method, a direct transvitreal approach is required; in the absence of vitreous haemorrhage, the foreign body is visible and its relation to the retina can be established.

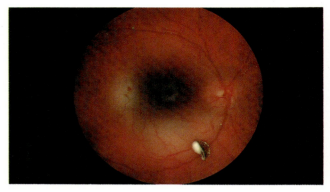

Fig.9.13 Small steel foreign body lying in front of the retina.

If the particle is free in the vitreous, there is a high risk of siderosis and early removal is indicated. An infusion line is prepared and removal is accomplished via the pars plana with intravitreal forceps; various instruments are available for this (see Fig. 7.8), and those with cup-shaped or flat blades are the most suitable for grasping a foreign body.

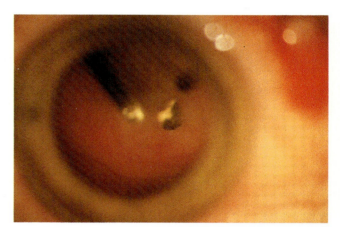

Fig.9.14 The same foreign body seen with the fibreoptic light system during transvitreal removal.

If a small steel foreign body has impacted posteriorly,the risks of siderosis are less as it may encapsulate, while the risks of removal are greater, as this involves manipulations on the surface of the retina. Deeply embedded or subretinal particles are observed for evidence of siderosis before proceeding. A foreign body exposed on the inner surface of the retina is likely to produce siderosis and should be removed.

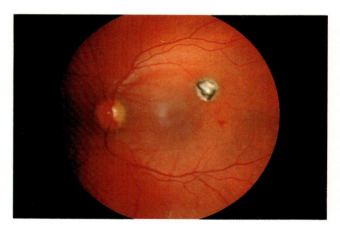

Fig.9.15 An impacted foreign body exposed on the surface of the retina near the macula.

The foreign body is approached across the vitreous, and the surrounding membrane is split across the surface of the particle using a fibreoptic pick or disposable needle bent at the tip. The foreign body is then gently mobilised and, once free, it can be removed with forceps.

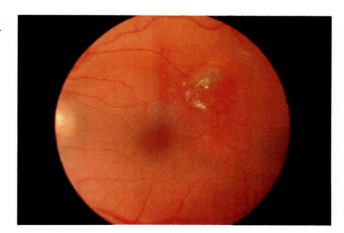

Fig.9.16 The appearance one week after removal, showing the reaction in the bed of the foreign body.

Posterior foreign bodies obscured by haemorrhage

Steel foreign bodies that have impacted posteriorly form the commonest group of injuries with failed magnetic extraction; these are often associated with dense vitreous haemorrhage. X-ray localisation (see page 6.20) and CAT scanning can establish whether the foreign body is still in the eye. Surgery is indicated both to remove the foreign body and prevent intraocular fibrosis. In the absence of an acute inflammatory reaction or deteriorating retinal function, surgery is deferred for two to four weeks to minimise the risk of secondary haemorrhage. Non-magnetic particles present with a similar problem: they have usually resulted from an explosion injury, with a large ragged fragment causing extensive internal damage. Copper fragments or its alloys cause a severe inflammatory response and early surgery will be needed, but other metals are less reactive and surgery is deferred until there is less risk of secondary bleeding.

Anterior removal

Injuries from large ragged fragments have often ruptured the lens, and these patients will have undergone lensectomy and anterior vitrectomy at the time of primary repair. The infusion line needs to be inserted away from the area of damage, and an irrigating contact lens is helpful in a traumatised eye where continued capillary bleeding from the conjunctiva can be a problem. Once the organising haemorrhage has been removed, an encapsulated foreign body may be visible, impacted in the posterior retina.

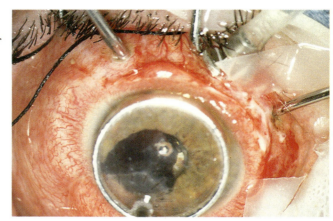

Fig.9.17 Secondary vitrectomy for removal of an aluminium fragment: primary repair included lensectomy and anterior vitrectomy.

If the particle has ricocheted internally, it is usually found in the vitreous cortex inferiorly and is mobilised during the vitrectomy. Once free, the foreign body can be grasped with intraocular forceps prior to removal.

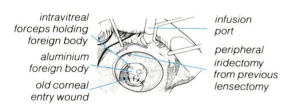

intravitreal forceps holding foreign body
aluminium foreign body
old corneal entry wound
infusion port
peripheral iridectomy from previous lensectomy

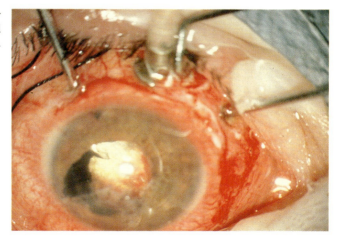

Fig.9.18 Aluminium foreign body mobilised and brought forwards with intraocular forceps.

In an aphakic eye, a large foreign body is removed via the anterior segment. After closing the ports with scleral plugs, a limbal incision is prepared and sutures are placed, which are tied temporarily while the foreign body is brought forwards. The foreign body is then extracted via the anterior segment and the limbal wound is secured.

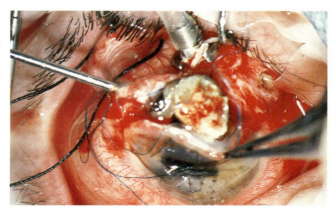

Fig.9.19 Removal of the foreign body through the anterior segment.

Further posterior segment surgery is required for the consequences of intraocular fibrosis (see page 9.13). Despite the severity of injury, if retinal detachment can be prevented, the eye settles well with retention of some vision. Acuity is usually poor because of damage to the macular region.

9.7

Pars plana removal

If the lens is intact, a pars plana extraction is performed. When the foreign body has been mobilised, one of the sclerotomies is enlarged with a blade, followed by bipolar cautery to the uvea, which can then be cut with fine scissors. Sutures are placed for closure of the sclerotomy after extraction.

The sclerotomy must be large enough to allow easy removal of the foreign body, otherwise tissue may be dragged into the wound, or the foreign body may be dropped. A further enlargement may be needed during removal as it is difficult to judge the size of large, ragged particles.

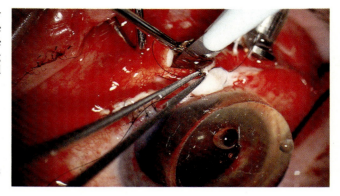

Fig.9.20 Enlarging a sclerotomy for removal of a large brass foreign body (note repaired entry wound at the limbus).

The foreign body may slip from the grip of the intraocular forceps which have a weak indirect action, and removal is aided by using direct action forceps which grip more firmly. The assistant helps during removal by holding sclerotomy open with forceps.

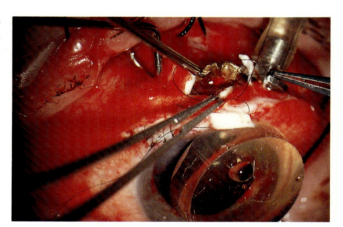

Fig.9.21 Assisting the extraction of a brass foreign body.

The infusion line is kept half-open during removal, to prevent collapse of the globe once the foreign body is free of the wound. Before closure, the sclerotomy is carefully cleaned and any tags of tissue are abscised.

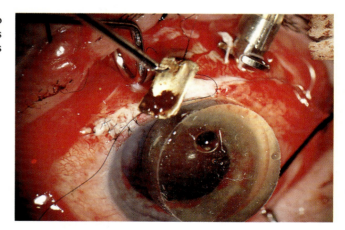

Fig.9.22 A large brass foreign body removed via the pars plana incision.

Extensive retinal damage is often present, and the severity of changes may require the use of intravitreal silicone oil (see page 9.13), to prevent retinal detachment in the postoperative period.

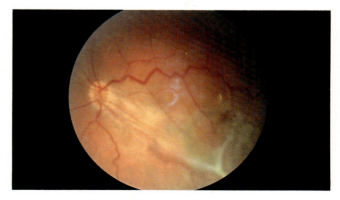

Fig.9.23 Extensive posterior segment damage and preretinal fibrosis after removal of an intraocular foreign body.

Retained Intraocular Foreign Bodies

The term 'retained' intraocular foreign body should be reserved for those patients presenting with the late complications associated with metallosis. These injuries are due to small particles that cause minimal symptoms at the time of injury. If not detected at the time and no acute inflammatory episode occurs, then the patient rarely presents before six months have elapsed, and sometimes the time interval can be several years. The retained metallic particle slowly oxidises with release of metallic ions: steel particles release ferric ions (unless in a protected environment like the lens), and this results in siderosis. Particles containing a small amount of copper release cupric ions, resulting in chalcosis. The latter is extremely rare, but less damaging to vision than siderosis.

Retained Steel Foreign Bodies

The retention of a steel fragment within the eye leads to various changes associated with the release of ferric ions. Irreversible damage to intracellular enzyme systems occurs, with deposition of insoluble compounds. The distribution of ferric compounds depends on the position of the foreign body: a retained fragment in the anterior segment will cause early deposition of iron in the iris, ciliary body and lens epithelium; the retinal pigment epithelium and inner layers of the retina are affected later.

A retained fragment in the posterior segment affects retinal function early; the iron compounds are transported to the outer layers of the retina by Muller's fibres. The vitreous becomes highly degenerate, often leading to rhegmatogenous retinal detachment.

Anterior segment involvement

One of the earliest symptoms is loss of accommodation; the patient may notice a brown discolouration of the iris or dilation of the pupil. The intraocular pressure can be low from damage to the ciliary epithelium, or raised because of iron-laden macrophages in the trabecular meshwork. Rust spots develop in the lens epithelium, forming a ring at the pupil margin.

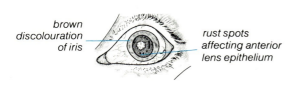

brown discolouration of iris — rust spots affecting anterior lens epithelium

Fig.9.24 Siderosis of the anterior segment.

Posterior segment involvement

Siderosis involving the retina can be well advanced before any visible changes occur; the early symptoms include night blindness and loss of peripheral field, but the patient is frequently unaware of any visual disturbance. Scattered pigmentation develops in the retina, which is most pronounced close to the foreign body, and the vitreous becomes degenerate and syneretic.

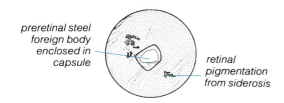

preretinal steel foreign body enclosed in capsule — retinal pigmentation from siderosis

Fig.9.25 Siderosis of the retina around a preretinal foreign body.

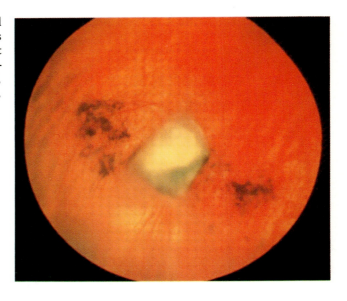

Other presentations

One of the commonest presentations is from a *rhegmatogenous retinal detachment* due to the associated vitreous degeneration; 50% of patients with retained particles present in this way. The retinal detachment results in sudden loss of vision that draws attention to the problem. The retinal tear is typically an equatorial horseshoe break or giant retinal tear unrelated to the position of the foreign body, although in some cases transgel traction is also present.

Recurrent uveitis is also common in an eye with a retained foreign body; this may be associated with disc and macular oedema, which can confuse the diagnosis.

Diagnosis and localisation

In established siderosis, the clinical picture is quite characteristic; the eye should be carefully examined for evidence of a penetrating wound or a track through iris and lens. There are two common sites for retained particles: firstly in the ciliary body following entry through a limbal wound, and secondly in the inferior vitreous adjacent to the pars plana or peripheral retina after passing through cornea and lens. The drainage angle should be examined with the gonioscope, and the peripheral retina checked with scleral indentation.

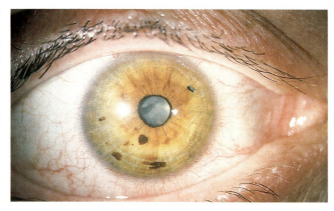

Fig.9.26 Hole in the iris and a mature cataract in a patient with a retained ciliary body particle.

X-rays are not always positive, as the particle may have lost much of its metallic nature; bone-free x-rays may be helpful in this situation. Peripheral retinal foreign bodies are often visible, particularly with indentation, but those anterior to the ora serata cannot easily be seen. The electroacoustic locator (using the most sensitive probe) will help confirm the position.

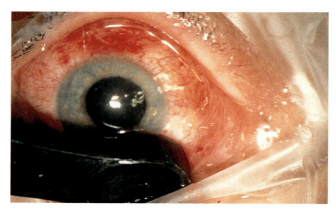

Fig.9.27 Confirming a retained foreign body in the ciliary body, using the electroacoustic locator.

Visual acuity is often well preserved until the late stages, but the visual field shows marked constriction. The diagnosis is confirmed by electrodiagnostic testing, and the earliest changes will be seen in dark adaptation and the electro-oculogram.

As the condition progresses, the electroretinogram becomes affected. Initially there is a supernormal response with loss of the oscillatory potentials, which is followed by a progressive reduction in the B-wave until it is extinguished.

The electroretinogram will also be affected by a rhegmatogenous retinal detachment, so the interpretation will be difficult in patients with both conditions.

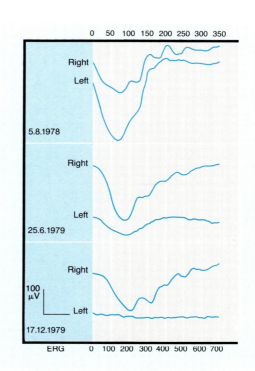

Fig.9.28 Serial electroretinograms showing progressive reduction in function with a retained steel foreign body in the left eye (surgery refused).

Management

Once siderosis is advanced, removal of the retained particle may not prevent progression; in fact, disturbance of the particle during surgery may potentiate the damage. If the electroretinogram is reduced by 50% or more, a poor outcome is to be expected. If the changes are early, serial retinal function tests should be performed: if there is evidence of progression, the foreign body should be removed.

Although the approach is similar to that described for fresh foreign bodies, certain important differences must be borne in mind: the foreign body will have lost much of its magnetism and may be difficult to locate on x-ray; if the foreign body cannot be seen, the ciliary body is the most likely site. Preoperative assessment with the electroacoustic locator confirms both the location and the presence of residual iron; surgery should not be attempted without a positive localisation.

With retained fragments, the particle will be encapsulated and fibrosed with adhesion to adjacent structures. A direct external approach is used only for particles anterior to the equator; since the vitreous is highly degenerate and the surgery will involve entry to the vitreous cavity, *an infusion line via the pars plana is essential* in all cases. Without this, the globe collapses and the foreign body can disappear from view. Having localised the foreign body, a double trapdoor is prepared as described earlier (page 6.23). The particle may be felt when the uveal tissue is incised, and often presents in the wound, enabling removal with fine forceps; alternatively, a powerful electromagnet is used for the extraction.

Foreign bodies at or posterior to the equator will need transvitreal removal as described earlier (page 9.6). Attempted transcleral removal will result in retinal incarceration. These injuries have a high risk of retinal detachment and all cases should have an encirclement of the vitreous base and appropriate buckling procedures.

If the visual impairment is due to a siderotic lens, cataract extraction is justifiable. An intracapsular extraction is the procedure of choice, because of the iron deposition within the lens epithelium.

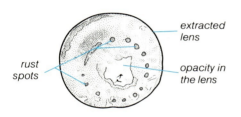

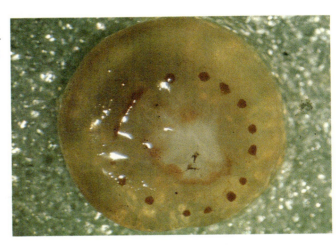

Fig.9.29 Siderotic lens extracted, showing rust spots.

Prevention of siderosis

When a decision is made not to attempt removal of a posteriorly impacted foreign body, the risk of siderosis may be reduced by restricting the adjacent blood supply and limiting the oxidation of the particle. A ring of laser therapy is applied around the site of the foreign body to create an avascular scar. Serial retinal function tests will be required to monitor the condition.

Systemic treatment with chelating agents has not proved helpful in the management of retained foreign bodies. Iron chelation cannot reverse established siderosis, and surgery is more effective in the early cases.

Rhegmatogenous retinal detachment

If the patient presents with a rhegmatogenous retinal detachment associated with a retained intraocular foreign body, the management is difficult: surgery to replace the detachment combined with removal of the intraocular foreign body is likely to fail; rapid pre-retinal fibrosis often develops, accompanied by rubeosis iridis, leading to a painful blind eye and ultimately enucleation.

The retinal problem should be tackled first on its own merits. If successful reattachment is achieved, the degree of siderosis can be assessed over a period of time, monitoring the recovery (if any) of the electroretinogram and visual field. Siderotic changes are likely to be advanced, and in most patients the retained particle is best left undisturbed.

Retained Copper Foreign Bodies

Only a small fragment containing little copper will produce chalcosis, as larger fragments cause a severe endophthalmitis in the early stages. Cupric ions differ from ferric ions by not penetrating within the cells; instead, they become deposited in basement membranes. As with siderosis, the degenerative vitreous changes may lead to rhegmatogenous retinal detachment; this will be the main indication for surgical intervention. Unless easily accessible, a retained copper-containing foreign body should be left alone.

Chalcosis has a variable effect on vision, and the course of this condition may cover many years. In some cases the electroretinogram is affected, while in others it remains normal for years. Eventually, cupric deposits on the lens may give rise to visual impairment.

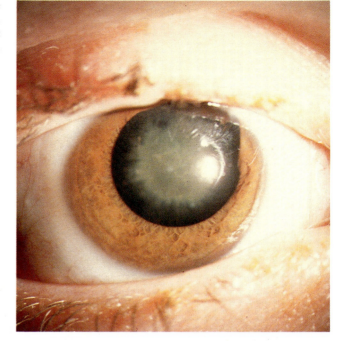

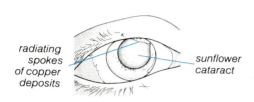

radiating
spokes
of copper
deposits

sunflower
cataract

Fig.9.30 Sunflower cataract in chalcosis.

A beautiful metallic sheen is present in Descemet's membrane and on the anterior and posterior lens capsule; glistening deposits are seen in the vitreous, which may be deposited on the internal limiting membrane in front of the macula.

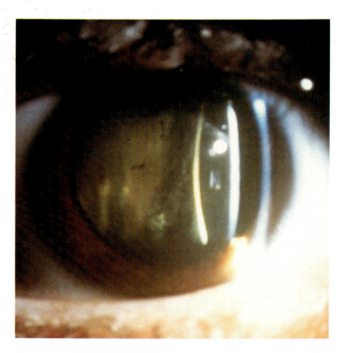

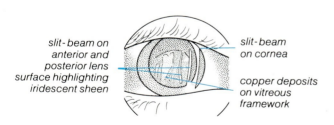

slit-beam on
anterior and
posterior lens
surface highlighting
iridescent sheen

slit-beam
on cornea

copper deposits
on vitreous
framework

Fig.9.31 Slit-lamp view showing lens deposits and vitreous change.

Retinal Complications after a Posterior Segment Perforation

Retinal incarceration

This may complicate scleral lacerations either because of incomplete penetration, or following an injury accompanied by contusion such as an air-gun pellet. If retinal incarceration is noted at the time of primary repair, a pars plana infusion line should be set up after temporary closure of the wound. If possible a vitrectomy is then carried out, freeing the incarceration internally. Often internal bleeding prevents this, and the wound should be thoroughly cleaned with the cutter externally. The posterior segment should be distended with air at the end of surgery, and the wound supported with a scleral silicone sponge after applying cryotherapy.

Gross retinal incarceration in a penetrating wound stimulates rapid epiretinal fibrosis leading to progressive retinal detachment. Reconstructive surgery is often unsuccessful and may lead to a degenerate eye, so it is only attempted in desperate cases where both eyes have been injured. Surgery should be limited to removing vitreous traction, accompanied by an encirclement and support to the incarceration site. Internal tamponade should not be used as this will produce retinal dialyses, nor should the incarceration be distrubed as this will precipitate a severe inflammatory reaction.

Minor degrees of retinal incarceration can complicate intraocular foreign bodies at sites of impaction or ricochet; this can be made worse by extracting large foreign bodies through the retina, particularly if

removal has been delayed. A transvitreal approach helps avoid this (see page 9.6), although epiretinal fibrosis remains a common complication.

When extensive retinal damage is present, internal tamponade is used to prevent detachment from epiretinal fibrosis. After preliminiary vitrectomy and division of fibrotic bands, silicone oil (1,000 cs viscosity) is exchanged via the infusion line using a flute needle to expel the intraocular saline by hydrostatic pressure. Manual injection requires considerable pressure and, if available, a mechanical pump facilitates this; care must be taken not to overfill the globe particularly in phakic eyes, as lens dislocation may occur.

After closing the vitrectomy ports, the state of the retina is then re-assessed, followed by external support and cryotherapy to the edge of the retinal break.

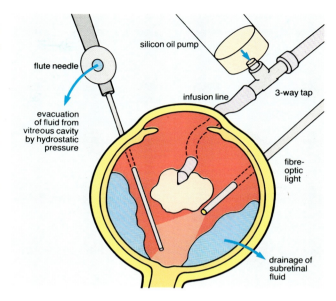

Fig.9.32 Diagram illustrating silicone oil exchange.

Peripheral fibrosis after penetrating trauma

Vitrectomy is not always required when an anterior scleral laceration has resulted in minimal vitreous haemorrhage and only localised fibrosis. Peripheral retinal elevation can develop after several months and should be supported locally; the laceration is usually running posteriorly, and a radial silicone sponge counteracts the adjacent traction. Cryotherapy should be

applied to the vitreous base in the quadrant affected by the wound. An encirclement is required if the retinal detachment is more extensive. (This procedure is always carried out when vitrectomy is performed for established intraocular fibrosis, as traction on the vitreous base has often led to small oral breaks).

Retinal tears

Extensive corneo-scleral perforations with expulsion of intraocular contents can be complicated by retinal dialyses resulting in giant tear formation with folding of the retina. The management is similar to those arising from closed eye injuries (see below).

Rhegmatogenous retinal detachment is another

common presentation of siderosis (see page 9.11); the tears result from vitreous degeneration and are not usually caused by traction. Conventional retinal surgery is carried out first without attempting to remove the foreign body; retinal function is then evaluated before considering extraction.

Retinal Tears Complicating Closed Eye Injuries

Blunt injury to the eye may result in peripheral retinal damage leading to retinal detachment (see page 5.15): limbal or anterior scleral impacts can lead to a retinal dialysis, while more posterior damage causes large round retinal tears or choroidal ruptures. Retinal dialyses are the commonest problem, and those that are less than $90°$ (see Fig.5.25) should respond favourably to conventional surgery.

After applying cryotherapy to the edges of the break,

the tear is sealed with a tangential 3 mm silicone sponge. At the two extremities, the mattress sutures need to be placed very anteriorly (one limb often needs to be in front of a muscle insertion), otherwise the indentation will be posterior to the tear; additional sutures are placed over the apex of the tear to increase the indentation. Drainage of subretinal fluid is not normally required for fresh cases, but if the retinal detachment is long-standing, drainage behind the indentation is performed.

Giant retinal tears

Retinal dialyses over 90% have a better prognosis than giant equatorial breaks, as the vitreous is attached to the posterior edge of the tear. If there is no subretinal fluid, cryotherapy to both edges of tear is sufficient, but if detached, vitrectomy with internal tamponade and external indentation will be required.

Minor trauma is often implicated in giant equatorial

tears, but pre-existing vitreoretinal degeneration is the major factor. The vitreous is attached to the anterior edge of the tear, while the posterior edge is free to fall over. Surgery is complicated and involves pars plana vitrectomy as well as internal tamponade with a 60/40 mixture of air and sulphur hexafluoride gas or silicone oil (1,000 cs viscosity).

If silicone oil is used, removal is usually carried out within six months to reduce the incidence of cataract, providing there is no equatorial fibrosis; in aphakic eyes, silicone oil in the anterior chamber may cause endothelial damage, or emulsify, causing silicone droplets in the anterior chamber; this can lead to raised intraocular pressure, and is an indication for removal.

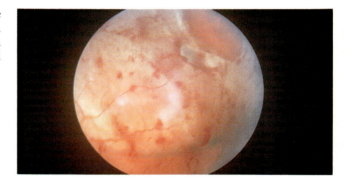

Fig.9.33 'Inverse hypopyon' from silicone oil emulsification in the anterior chamber.

Ragged equatorial retinal breaks

These are usually the result of direct mechanical damage from a posterior scleral impact and are associated with widespread retinal oedema; spontaneous pigmentation creating adhesion can occur, but progressive retinal detachment sometimes develops.

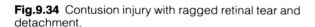

Fig.9.34 Contusion injury with ragged retinal tear and detachment.

They are awkward retinal breaks to treat because of their large circular shape: the Lincoff balloon technique can be helpful in this situation as it produces a wide smooth indentation. It consists of a fine self-retaining catheter which is distended during surgery with sterile saline.

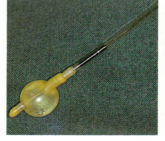 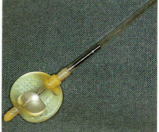

Fig.9.35 left & right The Lincoff balloon showing expansion of the tip with sterile saline.

The technique involves cryotherapy to the retinal tear, then the tip of the catheter is passed through a small conjunctival incision, and the latex balloon is slowly inflated. The position of the indentation and the patency of the central retinal artery are monitored with the indirect ophthalmoscope. When inflation is complete and the position satisfactory, the conjunctival entry wound is sutured around the catheter to stabilise it.

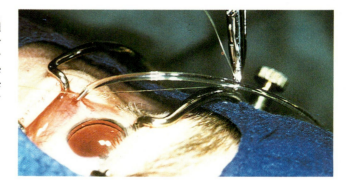

Fig.9.36 Lincoff balloon secured in position over an irregular retinal tear.

Although this has proved successful in some cases, our experience with this technique has been generally disappointing as the position and size of the indentation is not always maintained, and marked tissue reaction occurs making any subsequent surgery difficult.

Apart from this technique, cryotherapy and conventional external indentation with a large silicone sponge may be feasible, or if the tear is too large, vitrectomy combined with air exchange and posturing in the postoperative period is carried out.

Peripheral choroidal ruptures

These also follow a direct blow over the sclera, and may coexist with ragged retinal tears; typically there are multiple eliptical splits in both the choroid and retina, with extensive underlying haemorrhage. The reaction that follows the choroidal damage and subretinal haemorrhage is usually sufficient to create dense retinal adhesion, but occasionally retinal detachment can occur, requiring conventional retinal surgery.

10

The Management of Late Extraocular Complications

LATE COMPLICATIONS AFFECTING EYELID FUNCTION AND LACRIMAL DRAINAGE

In this section, the late complications affecting eyelid function and lacrimal drainage will be described and appropriate treatment outlined; the surgical techniques will not be discussed in detail, and reference should be made to standard texts on Ophthalmic Plastic Surgery.

In general, secondary surgery for complications resulting from cicatrisation should be delayed if possible for at least six months, to allow the scar tissue to mature and become less hyperplastic; however, earlier intervention is needed if there is severe corneal exposure.

In injuries resulting from a bony deformity, liaison with a maxillofacial surgeon is helpful.

Traumatic Ptosis from a Damaged Levator Aponeurosis

The majority of traumatic ptoses will recover after a careful primary repair of an injury to the upper lid. Persisting ptosis can result from a retained foreign body (see page 2.7) and if suspected, these injuries should be explored early. Otherwise, a six month period should elapse before intervening, to allow for spontaneous recovery.

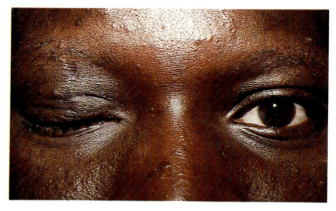

Fig.10.1 Persisting ptosis following an upper lid laceration. By courtesy of Mr. J.R.O. Collin.

If there is no improvement, the levator aponeurosis is explored from an anterior approach, preferably under local anaesthesia in order that the patient can co-operate during surgery to help identify the dehiscence in the aponeurosis.

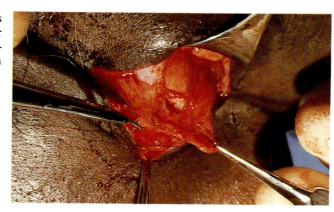

Fig.10.2 Exploration of the above patient revealed a dehiscence of the levator aponeurosis. By courtesy of Mr. J.R.O. Collin.

Once identified, the levator aponeurosis is plicated or secured to the superior border of the tarsal plate, followed by repair of the overlying skin wound. An improved cosmetic appearance with good lid elevation and adequate lid closure can be achieved with this technique.

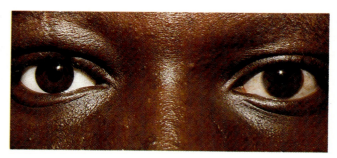

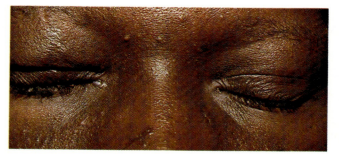

Fig.10.3 upper & lower Postoperative appearance after advancing and repairing the aponeurotic defect, showing good eyelid closure. By courtesy of Mr. J.R.O. Collin.

Corneal exposure from cicatricial ectropion causes discomfort and inflammation of the affected eye, with a risk of secondary infection. In ophthalmic practice the most common cause is contracture of a vertical laceration that has involved full-thickness eyelid tissue; this results in a V-shaped deformity of the affected eyelid, which impairs blinking and prevents adequate lid closure during sleep.

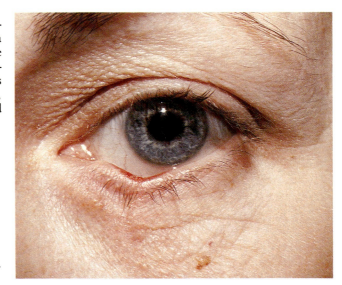

Fig.10.4 Lower lid cicatricial ectropion. By courtesy of Mr. J.R.O. Collin.

A localised deformity of the lid margin is corrected by a small full-thickness lid resection followed by repair of the eyelid (see page 2.5). If the scar extends vertically beyond the eyelid into the cheek or brow region, the scar is excised and a lengthening procedure carried out by performing multiple small z-plasties. After mobilising the triangular skin flaps (a–d), these are transposed horizontally to the apices (a_1–d_1), and sutured in position.

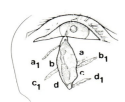

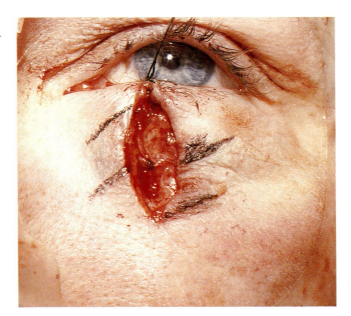

Fig.10.5 Excision of scar and skin marking for planned double z-plasty. By courtesy of Mr. J.R.O. Collin.

This technique breaks up the line of the scar and reduces the risk of further contracture. The technique can be applied to the cheek or brow region where there is room to mobilise tissues. If this is not possible (i.e. near the inner canthus), additional skin must be provided by a rotation flap or free graft, as appropriate.

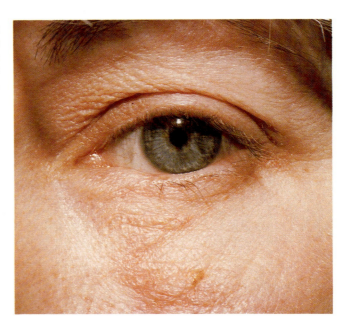

Fig.10.6 Postoperative appearance. By courtesy of Mr. J.R.O. Collin.

Full-thickness skin loss can also lead to contractures causing ectropion; this occurs rapidly after facial burns involving the eyelids and early skin grafting is required (see page 4.14). Less commonly this complication follows tissue loss from an injury such as a dog bite, and if grafting is not carried out at primary repair, contracture will result.

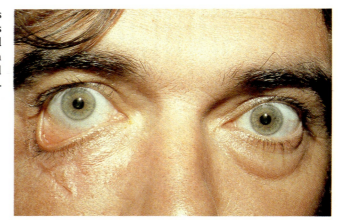

Fig.10.7 Cicatricial ectropion from skin loss. By courtesy of Mr. J.R.O. Collin.

This is corrected by excision of the scar and restoring the tissue defect with a free skin graft; suitable tissue can be obtained from the opposite upper lid or retro-auricular region. When the lateral aspect of the lower lid is affected the defect can be replaced by a cheek rotation flap.

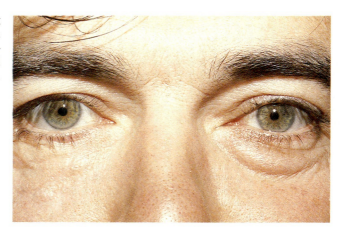

Fig.10.8 Postoperative appearance after full-thickness skin graft. By courtesy of Mr. J.R.O. Collin.

Cicatricial Entropion

Molten metal burns can cause extensive lid destruction with obliteration of the fornices and symblepharon leading to entropion and tethering of the globe. Involvement of the medial canthus can destroy the lacrimal passages. Inadequate protection of the cornea or damage from aberrant lashes causes chronic keratitis.

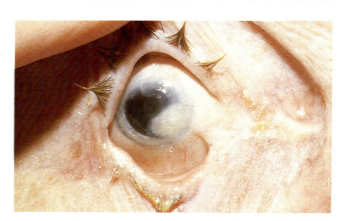

Fig.10.9 Destruction of the inner canthus after a molten metal burn, with tethering and cicatricial entropion with chronic keratitis. By courtesy of Mr. J.R.O. Collin.

If the problem is confined to a few aberrant lashes, epilation or cryoablation with an oculoplastic probe can control the condition, but if extensive symblepharon and entropion are present, surgical reconstruction is indicated. Conjunctival shrinkage or tethering is corrected by a mucous membrane graft, using conjunctiva from the upper fornix of the uninjured eye if this is available, or alternatively buccal mucous membrane. Although initially successful, further contracture often occurs, which should be allowed for at the time of surgery.

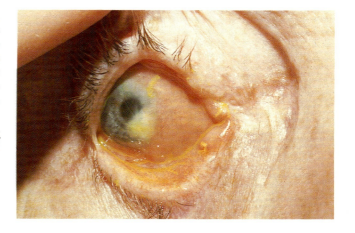

Fig.10.10 Postoperative appearance immediately after mucous membrane grafting showing improved abduction. By courtesy of Mr. J.R.O. Collin.

In this type of injury, extensive obliteration of the canaliculi is present and anatomical reconstruction is not possible. Troublesome epiphora is overcome by a conjunctivo-cysto-rhinostomy, with a lacrimal by-pass tube.

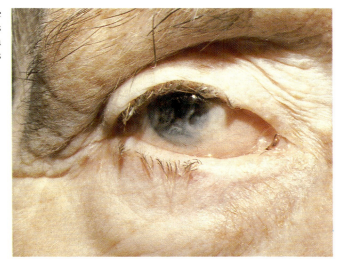

Fig.10.11 Late appearance of this injury after the insertion of a lacrimal by-pass tube. By courtesy of Mr. J.R.O. Collin.

Late Treatment of Damage to the Lacrimal Drainage Apparatus

Lacerations involving one canaliculus rarely result in troublesome epiphora, provided an accurate lid repair is carried out without disturbing the common canaliculus; damage to both canaliculi and the lacrimal sac is unusual as an isolated injury, but can occur from a deep laceration involving the inner canthal region. If the medial ligament has also been disrupted, the inner canthus is displaced laterally with a rounded configuration. This appearance is more commonly seen after a naso-orbital fracture (see page 3.9), from lateral displacement of the bony attachments of the medial ligament.

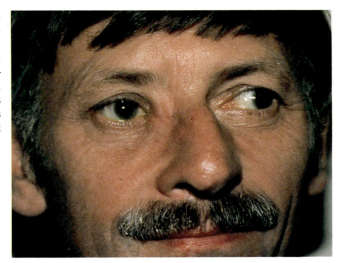

Fig.10.12 Disinsertion of the medial ligament and a mucocele of the lacrimal sac after a naso-orbital fracture.

If both canaliculi are damaged at the entrance to the lacrimal sac, a dacryo-cysto-rhinostomy is performed, with intubation of the canaliculi using silicone tubing. If intubation is difficult, the exploration is carried laterally under microscopic control, using the medial ligament as a guide to the position of the canaliculi; the obliterated portion is excised and the patent ends anastomosed to the lacrimal sac (C-D.C.R.). If the inner canthus requires reconstruction, two small holes are drilled anterior to the rhinostomy to allow wiring of the medial ligament.

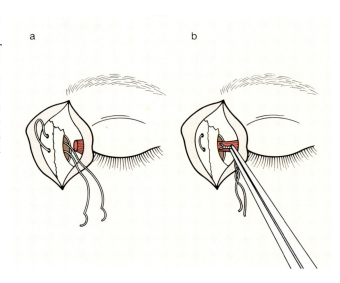

Fig.10.13 Diagram illustrating re-attachment of the medial ligament.

If an underlying bony deformity is present, reconstruction is best carried out by a maxillofacial surgeon. Late reconstruction often involves recreating the fracture followed by open repair with interosseous wiring. Obstruction to the nasolacrimal duct requires a dacryo-cysto-rhinostomy; if the bony deformity makes this impossible, a dacryocystectomy is performed including curettage of the nasolacrimal duct. This reduces the irritation from the chronic mucous discharge and the tendency to recurrent infection.

10.5

Blow-out fractures of the medial orbital wall rarely require either exploration or subsequent strabismus surgery, even if marked tethering is present initially; recovery to orthophoria with a full field of binocular single vision occurs spontaneously. With pure orbital floor fractures, approximately 10% of those with double vision initially will be left with troublesome diplopia requiring further strabismus surgery; these will almost all have undergone exploration and repair of the orbital floor in the early post-injury period, according to the criteria discussed in Chapter 3, page 3.5. A higher incidence of persisting diplopia occurs after repair of complex floor and zygomatic fractures.

If diplopia persists for several months after a blow-out fracture of the orbital floor, secondary strabismus surgery may be required. If the double vision only occurs on upgaze and the patient is orthophoric in the primary position and on downgaze, further intervention is inadvisable, as surgery may lead to more troublesome symptoms.

The most common problem requiring further treatment is a *hypotropia* in the primary position and restriction of movement of the affected eye on upgaze; less commonly a *hypertropia* is present with restriction on downgaze. Some patients are *orthophoric* in the primary position, but show marked restriction of both up- and downgaze with a very small field of binocular single vision.

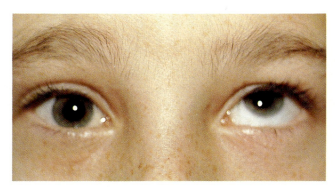

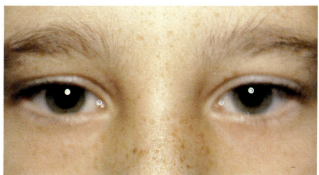

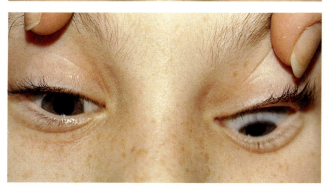

Fig.10.14 upper, middle, lower Orthophoria with persisting restriction of both up- and downgaze one month after repair of a right orbital floor fracture.

The blow-out fracture and subsequent repair of the orbital floor can lead to tethering of the sheath of the inferior rectus, muscle fibrosis from damage at the time of injury or during repair, or a neurogenic paresis. Duction tests (see page 3.4) help to confirm mechanical restrictions and fibrosis: the Hess chart and field of binocular single vision are helpful in assessing any improvement and identifying muscle sequelae (see page 3.5). Recovery occurs over several months and further surgery should not be undertaken until the condition has stabilised.

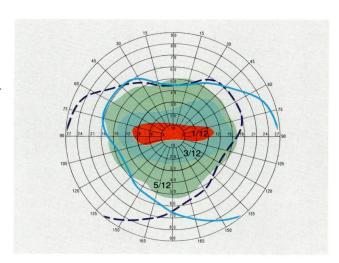

Fig.10.15 Serial fields of B.S.V. in the same patient showing full recovery of function over four months.

In many of these patients secondary muscle sequelae are not prominent in keeping with a mechanical restriction rather than a paresis or fibrosis. In most cases the deviation is purely vertical and surgery is directed at restoring binocular single vision in the primary position and on downgaze. As the results are not entirely predictable, the surgery is carried out in stages and an adjustable suture technique is used for muscle recessions (see page 10.6). With this technique larger recessions than is usual can be carried out, which can be adjusted the following day if necessary.

If a *hypotropia* is present in the primary position with mechanical restriction on upgaze, a recession of the affected inferior rectus (3 - 6 mm) is carried out. If there is no demonstrable passive restriction, the ipsilateral superior rectus is strengthened by resecting 3 - 5 mm; persisting hypotropia of the affected eye is further helped by recessing the contralateral superior rectus (3 - 6 mm).

If a *hypertropia* is present and there is weakness of the affected inferior rectus and overaction of the contralateral superior oblique muscle, a tenotomy of the latter is carried out. Alternatively, the paretic muscle can be strengthened by a resection (3 mm). Overaction of the ipsilateral superior rectus is unusual, but if present, the imbalance can be further helped by its recession (3 - 5 mm). After surgery, any residual inconcomitance on downgaze may require prismatic correction for reading.

Simultaneous ipsilateral recessions (4 - 6 mm) of both the inferior and superior rectus are helpful in those patients who are *orthophoric* in the primary position, but have restriction of the affected eye on both up- and downgaze (see Fig. 10.14); the adjustable suture technique is particularly useful in this situation, allowing orthophoria to be maintained. Some residual diplopia on extreme vertical gaze is likely.

Persisting Diplopia after Other Orbital Fractures

Supraorbital fractures (see page 3.10) are often associated with transient double vision from mechanical restriction due to haematoma formation. The orbital rim can be displaced and if not reduced early, it will leave a marked asymmetry of the facial appearance. Despite this, the diplopia usually resolves and a good field of binocular single vision is retained.

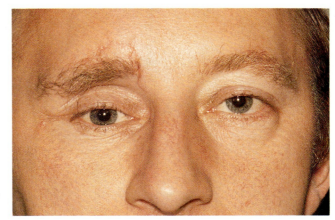

Fig.10.16 An old right supraorbital fracture with asymmetry but orthophoria.

Persisting diplopia can result from a depressed fracture with bony spicules, interfering with the function of the levator and superior rectus muscles; the limitation of eye movement is greatest on elevation in abduction and can be confused with the restriction following a blow-out fracture of the orbital floor. Exploration with elevation of the depressed fragment of bone is required.

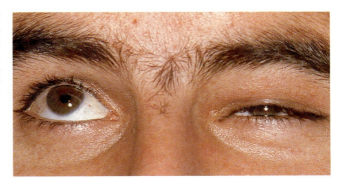

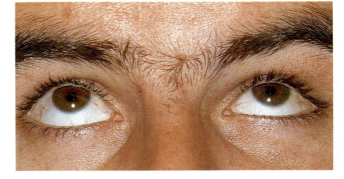

Fig.10.17 upper & lower A left supraorbital fracture six weeks after injury, showing fullness of the upper lid and restricted elevation; full recovery after refracturing and wiring the displaced supraorbital rim. By courtesy of Mr. M.J.C. Wake.

Persisting diplopia after other orbital fractures is unusual unless there has been damage to the cranial nerves; a third nerve palsy is common after the orbital apex syndrome (see page 3.14) and recovery is often incomplete. The management of this and other cranial nerve palsies is discussed later (see page 10.9).

Extensive naso-orbital fractures (see page 3.9) can be associated with damage to the medial rectus, but a persisting divergent squint is most often due to blindness from optic nerve damage (see Fig. 10.12: naso-orbital fracture and right divergence following optic nerve evulsion).

This technique is particularly useful in secondary strabismus surgery for late traumatic diplopia where surgery on the vertical muscles is often required; it allows larger recessions (up to 6 mm) to be carried out with more confidence. The technique has become possible because of the availability of fine, smooth, non-irritant sutures that are absorbable, such as 0.7 metric (6/0) polyglactin. The surgery is carried out under general anaesthesia, avoiding agents that will impair postoperative alertness, and the adjustment is made two to twenty-four hours later.

According to Jampolsky's technique, the conjunctiva is opened at the limbus and relaxed on each side of the muscle; after dividing the attachments of Tenon's capsule, a double-ended suture is locked to the insertion as shown, taking care to incorporate the posterior muscle sheath.

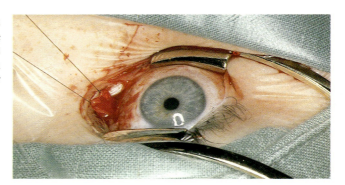

Fig.10.18 Placement of double-armed suture in the muscle insertion. By courtesy of Mr. H.E. Willshaw.

After separating the muscle, the two spatula needles are inserted from the point of minimum recession, passing obliquely within the sclera to exit close to the centre of the original insertion. The muscle is then allowed to fall back to the *maximum* recession required, so that the only postoperative adjustment will be an advancement if this proves necessary. The two suture ends are secured by a separate sliding triple knot formed with the same suture material. This is moved up and down the muscle sutures a few times to ensure that the knot moves freely.

Fig.10.19a,b,c Diagrams showing placement of sutures, final position of the recessed muscle, and the method of securing the adjustable suture.

The ends of all the sutures are kept long and left in the upper and lower fornices or taped onto the skin of the brow or cheek; those attached to the muscle are placed separately from those attached to the sliding knot. The conjunctiva is closed in a recessed position leaving access centrally for adjustment, and the eye is padded after instilling topical prednisolone and an antibiotic.

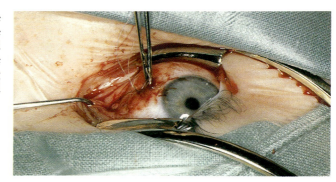

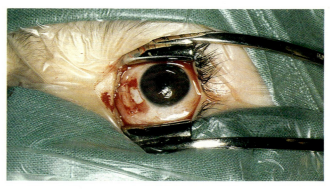

Fig.10.20 upper & lower Securing the suture ends of the recessed muscle and closure of the conjunctiva. By courtesy of Mr. H.E. Willshaw.

The following day the patient is seated upright and an orthoptic assessment is carried out; the adjustment is then made with the patient supine after applying 1% amethocaine drops. Occasionally a bradycardia results from the oculocardiac reflex and 0.6 mg of atropine should be available for injection if required. If the orthoptic assessment confirms that the position is satisfactory, the muscle suture is simply secured permanently and the ends trimmed.

If the recession has been too large, the muscle sutures are eased forwards through the point where they pass through the insertion, and countertraction is applied to the sliding knot; to perform this procedure the sutures are held with smooth tying forceps. The orthoptic assessment is then repeated and the suture secured when the position is satisfactory.

Late Treatment of Traumatic Third Nerve Palsies

Incomplete recovery after traumatic third nerve palsies can be complicated by ptosis, pupillary abnormalities and signs of aberrant regeneration (see page 3.16). Treatment is inadvisable for gross defects where diplopia is prevented by persisting ptosis, but if lid function recovers, troublesome double vision is often present, requiring further treatment. Secondary surgery for muscle imbalance is deferred for at least six months, to allow maximum recovery.

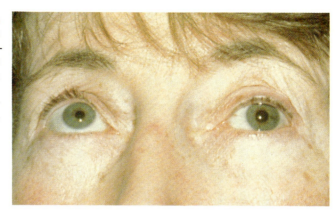

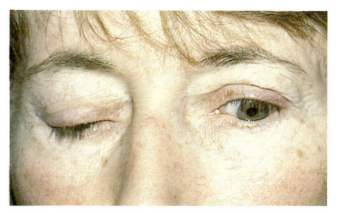

Fig.10.21 upper & lower Incomplete recovery of a left third nerve palsy, showing an exotropia with defective elevation and abnormal lid retraction on downgaze.

Surgical treatment

The exodeviation is corrected first: if this has become concomitant, bilateral horizontal surgery is performed first; subsequent surgery on the vertical component involves recession of overacting contralateral yoke muscles. Inappropriate lid elevation from misdirection is sometimes helped by a weakening operation or Faden procedure (see page 10.10) on the contralateral yoke muscle (right inferior rectus in the above example).

If a large-angle inconcomitant exotropia is present, surgery to the affected eye involves a full recession of the lateral rectus and a resection with advancement of the medial rectus: the latter is performed by securing each side of the muscle insertion in a clamp, then splitting the muscle longitudinally for about 10 mm; the globe is positioned in slight adduction and each slip of the medial rectus is secured 2 mm in front of the insertions of the superior and inferior rectus respectively, trimming off any excess.

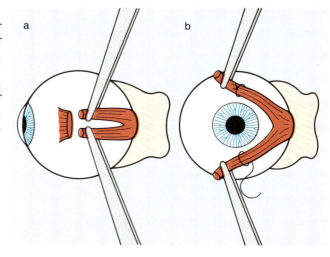

Fig.10.22 a, b Diagram showing technique for correction of a large exodeviation after a third nerve palsy.

10.9

Incomplete recovery of a sixth nerve palsy leaves an esotropia with horizontal diplopia which may be correctable with prisms or require surgical treatment.

A concomitant deviation is corrected by conventional horizontal surgery, but a large inconcomitant deviation with limited abduction is treated by recessing the ipsilateral medial rectus muscle and performing a muscle union operation (Jensen's procedure), or a transposition operation (Hummelsheim's operation) to strengthen the lateral rectus.

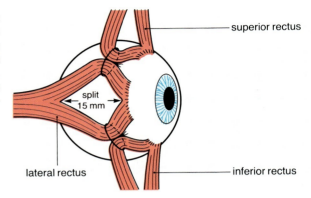

superior rectus

split 15 mm

lateral rectus

inferior rectus

The Jensen's procedure is most commonly performed; it involves splitting the superior and inferior rectus muscles and uniting the lateral halves to each half of the split lateral rectus tendon. A permanent suture (1 metric (5/0) braided polyester) is used, securing the slips approximately 12 mm back from the insertions; the suture should not be too tight, to avoid occluding the vascular supply.

Fig.10.23 Diagram illustrating the Jensen procedure.

Although this can improve the deviation in the primary position, abduction often remains defective and can be further improved by a recession or Faden operation on the contralateral medial rectus, depending on the residual angle. If an esophoria is still present, recession of the contralateral medial rectus is carried out, but if orthophoric, the Faden operation reduces the overaction of the yoke muscle without affecting the angle in the primary position.

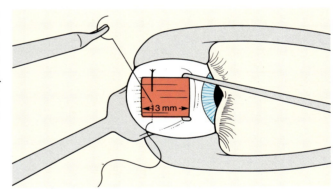

13 mm

Fig.10.24 Diagram illustrating the Faden operation.

Late Treatment of Traumatic Fourth Nerve Palsies

Initially these palsies give rise to a moderate vertical deviation and extorsion that can be partly compensated by a head tilt away from the affected side; tilting the head to the affected side increases the hypertropia.

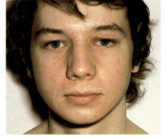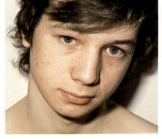

Fig.10.25 left & right Right superior oblique palsy after trauma, showing a right hypertropia when the head posture is abolished, and the typical head tilt adopted to compensate.

Recovery of the vertical deviation can occur, leaving a torsional defect that interferes with fusion. The adjustable Harada–Ito procedure is the treatment of choice, as it corrects the cyclodeviation without altering the vertical alignment. The procedure involves advancement of the anterior half of the superior oblique tendon to a position just above the lateral rectus insertion, using an adjustable suture technique. This is adjusted postoperatively using the double maddox rod test to eliminate any residual cyclodeviation.

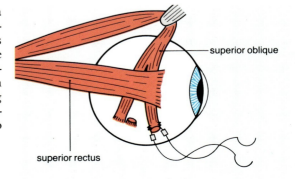

superior oblique

superior rectus

Fig.10.26 Diagram of the adjustable Harada-Ito procedure.

The vertical deviation, however, often persists. The choice of surgery will depend on the muscle sequelae following the superior oblique palsy, and the classification by Knapp into six groups based on the maximal hyperdeviation is helpful in planning the treatment. Surgery is best carried out in several stages.

Fig.10.27 Classification of pareses of the superior oblique muscle.

Class 1–3 deviations are the commonest problems encountered after a unilateral fourth nerve palsy.

Hypertropia of the affected eye:

1. greatest in abduction and elevation

2. greatest in abduction and depression

3. in abduction on both elevation and depression

4. as in 3, and on abduction and depression

5. in all depressed positions only

6. as in 2, with restricted elevation in adduction

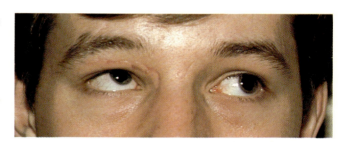

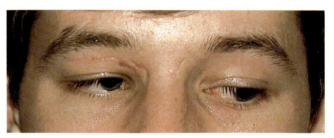

Fig.10.28 upper & lower Overaction of the right inferior oblique and weakness of the right superior oblique after trauma to the right orbital septum (cf.Fig.10.25).

Overaction of the ipsilateral inferior oblique muscle (class 1) is corrected by recessing it fully. If the deviation is greatest in the field of action of the paretic superior oblique muscle (class 2), plication of the superior oblique tendon is performed first. While this improves the deviation on depression, an acquired Brown's syndrome will be present on elevation. Alternatively, a recession of the contralateral inferior rectus is carried out.

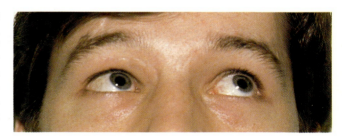

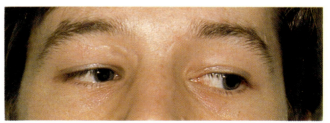

Fig.10.29 upper & lower Right superior oblique paresis improved by a recession of the ipsilateral inferior oblique, followed by a recession of the contralateral inferior rectus (c f. Fig.10.28).

Where the hypertropia spreads across the lower field in addition to the opposite side (class 4), or where the lower field only is affected (class 5), the surgery as described above for the vertical spread is carried out first. Where the lower field remains affected, further surgery is carried out if the hypertropia becomes greatest in the field of action of the ipsilateral inferior rectus; a resection of this muscle or a tenotomy of the contralateral superior oblique tendon is then performed.

In bilateral superior oblique palsies both tendons are plicated or advanced, with subsequent transposition of the medial rectus insertions by half a tendon's width downwards for a pronounced V pattern.

Where the superior oblique palsy is complicated by restriction of relaxation (Brown's syndrome – class 6), the tethering is freed first, using an absorbable gel-foam on the sclera to help prevent further adhesions and by keeping the globe in elevation in adduction with a traction suture taped to the forehead for several days. Secondary surgery for the superior oblique palsy is deferred until the condition is stable.

REHABILITATION AFTER INJURY

Difficulties with binocular vision
Persisting diplopia after injury often requires a protracted period of assessment before secondary surgery can be undertaken; if comfortable binocular single vision cannot be restored with prismatic correction, certain occupations such as working with machinery or on scaffolding are dangerous, and a prolonged period off work is required.

A similar situation arises after unilateral traumatic aphakia; although early correction with a daily wear soft contact lens can allow rapid rehabilitation, in many cases a hard contact lens is required, and time will be needed to increase the wearing time and assess tolerance. Many patients subsequently abandon contact lens wear because of discomfort or diplopia, but by this period they have usually adjusted to uniocular vision.

Blindness
Bilateral injury may result in partial or complete blindness; this is most likely to occur after severe chemical or thermal burns. It was also common after bilateral perforating injuries from windscreen accidents, but seat-belt legislation has almost abolished these injuries.

Loss of all useful vision in one eye
This will have serious implications for a person whose work demands stereoscopic vision. In industry, many firms will not allow a person to return to work on machinery, and although alternative employment with the firm is sometimes provided, this often means a drop in earning capacity. For young people embarking on a new career, certain occupations such as the Forces are precluded.

With regard to driving, if vision is completely normal in one eye there is no restriction on ordinary vehicles, but a heavy goods vehicle licence cannot be obtained. Young individuals adjust rapidly to loss of sight in one eye, but the elderly require a longer period of rehabilitation, and should be advised not to drive for three months.

Complete blindness causes a severe emotional disturbance, and a great deal of support is required; blind registration should be completed at an early stage to enable mobility training and rehabilitation to proceed.

COMPENSATION

Medicolegal claims frequently arise after injury at work, from assault, or following an automobile accident. A detailed history recorded on presentation is invaluable, as details can become confused with time; in particular, the wearing of protective safety goggles or seat-belt should be noted, as conflicting claims may be made at a later date. This will influence the level of compensation.

In some cases the injury contributes only partly to disability, such as retinal detachement developing after a head injury. When trauma is the sole cause of disability, protracted medicolegal claims tend to perpetuate symptoms which disappear when settlement is agreed. The period of incapacity, any loss of earnings or inability to carry on with occupations and recreations, and any permanent cosmetic or functional disability, should be taken into account. Complicated cases would require serial assessments over a long period.

Visual loss is measured in terms of acuity and visual field, and percentages are often requested; at best this can only be an estimate and functional impairment will depend on the nature of damage. For example, macular damage has a more profound effect on reading vision compared with distance acuity, while the opposite is true of damage affecting medial transparency. The importance of loss of stereoscopic vision despite good corrected acuity needs special emphasis, as this is a difficult concept for non-medical persons to understand.

Malingering is not uncommon after trivial injuries, and if there is doubt concerning the subjective level of vision other tests are used for an objective assessment, for example prism deviation, red-green glasses, the Catford drum acuity test, stereoscopic tests and VEP (page 3.15). The claim of complete blindness is easier to refute than partial loss of vision.

PREVENTION OF INJURIES

Seat-belt legislation has had a dramatic effect on the incidence of serious eye injuries following road traffic accidents. Much has also been done to reduce the incidence of industrial accidents by appropriate protective measures, but more publicity should be given to the use of similar goggles at home, as most mechanical injuries occur in the domestic situation. Any person admitted with a sporting injury should be advised on protection, and those wearing glasses should have toughened or plastic lenses for sport; this applies to those at risk from injury, such as children and epileptic patients.

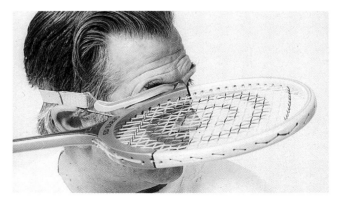

Fig.10.30 Protective goggles for squash players.

References

Chapter 1

Ocular injuries from liquid golf ball cores. D.R. Lucas, A.C. Dunham, W.R. Lee, W. Weir & F.C.F. Wilkinson, (1976) Brit. J. Ophthal. **60:**740-747.

Chapter 2

Primary repair of eyelid lacerations. H.K. Mehta, (1978) Trans. Ophthal. Soc. U.K. **98:**75-80.

Repair and reconstruction in the orbital region. J.C. Mustarde, (1980) Churchill Livingstone, 2nd edition.

Long-term review of injuries to the lacrimal drainage apparatus. Y.M. Canavan & D.B. Archer, (1979) Trans. Ophthal. Soc. U.K. **99:**201-204.

Chapter 3

Blow-out fracture of the orbit mechanism and correction of internal orbital fracture. B. Smith & W.F. Regan, (1957) Am. J. Ophthalmol. **44:**733-739.

Management of orbital floor fractures. J.M. Emery, G.K. von Noorden & D.A. Schlernitzauer, (1972) Am. J. Ophthalmol. **74:**299-306.

Non surgical management of blow-out fractures of the orbital floor. A.M. Putterman, T. Stevens & M.J. Urist, (1974) Am. J. Ophthalmol. **77:**232-239.

Long-term follow-up of orbital blow-out fractures with and without surgery. B. Dulley & P. Fells, (1975) Mod. Problem Ophthalmol. **14:**467-470.

Current Treatment of Blow-out Fractures. R.B. Wilkins & W.E. Havins, (1982) Ophthalmol. **89(5):**464-466.

A case of isolated medial wall fracture with medial rectus entrapment following seemingly trivial trauma. R.G. Mirsky & R.A. Saunders, (1979) J. Paediatric Ophthalmol. **16:**287-290.

Repair and reconstruction in the orbital region. J.C. Mustarde, (1980) 2nd edn., p. 245; published by Churchill Livingstone.

Primary treatment of naso-ethmoid injuries with increased intercanthal distance. M.F. Stranc, (1970) Brit. J. Plastic Surg. **23:**8-25.

Naso-orbital Fractures, Complications and Treatment. C.K. Beyer, R.L. Fabian & B. Smith, (1982) Ophthalmol. **89(5):**456-463.

Orbital roof fractures: neurologic and neurosurgical considerations. J.C. Flanagan, D.L. McLachlan & G.M. Shannon, (1980) Ophthalmol. **87:**325-329.

Diagnosis and management of a wooden orbital foreign body: case report. J.A. Macrae, (1979) Brit. J. Ophthal. **63:**848-851.

The orbital puncture wound: intracranial complications of a retained foreign body. E.L. Kazarian, N.A. Stokes & J.T. Flynn, (1980) J. Paediatric Ophthalmol. **17:**247-250.

Subperiosteal haematomas of the orbit in young males: a serious complication of trauma or surgery in the eye region. J.R. Wolter, (1979) Trans. Am. Ophth. Soc. **77:**104-115.

Computed tomography in the management of orbital trauma. A.S. Grove Jr., (1982) Ophthalmol. **89(5):**433-440.

Transantral-Ethmoidal Decompression of Optic Canal Fracture. J.S. Kennerdell, G.A. Amsbaugh & E.N. Myers, (1976) Arch. Ophthalmol. **94:**1040-1043.

Visual prognosis of traumatic optic nerve damage. H. Matsuzaki, (1981) Acta. Soc. Ophthalmol. Jpn. **85:**824-836.

The orthoptic role in head injuries. J. Mein, (1980-81) Aust. Orthopt. J. **18:**10-14.

Ischaemic ocular necrosis from carotid-cavernous fistula. W.H. Spencer, H.S. Thompson & W.F. Hoyt, (1973) Brit. J. Ophthal. **57:**145-152.

Ophthalmic manifestations of the battered baby syndrome. B. Harcourt & D. Hopkins, (1971) Brit. Med. J. **3:**398-401.

Purtscher's retinopathy related to chest compression by safety belts. J.S. Kelly, (1972) Amer. J. Ophthal. **74:**278-283.

Ocular complications of lightning. L.P. Noel, W.N. Clarke & D. Addison, (1980) J. Paediatric Ophthalmol. **17:**245-246.

Eclipse retinopathy. S.P. Dhir, A. Gupta & I.S. Jain, (1981) Brit. J. Ophthal. **65(1):**42-45.

Chapter 4

Thermal and chemical burns. M.J. Roper-Hall, (1965) Trans. Ophthal. Soc. U.K. **85:**631-646.

Eye injuries from car battery explosions. A.T. Moore, H. Cheng & D.L. Boase, (1982) Brit. J. Ophthal. **66:**141-144.

Treatment of the alkali-burned cornea. S.I. Brown, M.P. Tragakis & D.B. Pearce, (1972) Amer. J. Ophthal. **74:**316-320.

Irrigation of the anterior chamber for the treatment of alkali burns. R.P. Burns & C.E. Hikes, (1979) Amer. J. Ophthal. **88:**119-120.

Corneal transplantation for severe alkali burns. S.I. Brown, M.P. Tragakis & D.B. Pearce, (1972) Trans. Am. Acad. Ophthalmol. Otolaryngol. **76:**1266-1274.

A follow-up report on transplantation of the alkali-burned cornea. S.I. Brown, S.E. Bloomfield & D.B. Pearce, (1974) Amer. J. Ophthal. **77:**538-542.

Immunosuppression and selective inflammatory cell depletion. C.S. Foster, R.P. Zelt, T. Mai-Phan & K.R. Keynon, (1982) Arch. Ophthal. **100:**1820-1824.

Regulation of collagenase – therapeutic considerations. M. Berman, (1978) Trans. Ophthal. Soc. U.K., **98:**397-405.

Superoxide Radical Scavenging Agents in the treatment of Alkali Burns. V.S. Nirankari, S.D. Varma, V. Lakhanpal & R.D. Richards, (1981) Arch. Ophthal. **99:**886-887.

Ascorbic acid in the treatment of alkali burns of the eye. R.R. Pfister & C.A. Paterson, (1980) Ophthalmology (Rochester) **87:**1050-1057.

Corneal changes due to alkali burns. G. Renard, M. Hirsch & Y. Pouliquen, (1978) Trans. Ophthal. Soc. U.K., **98:**379-382.

Thermal burns: the management of thermal burns of the lids and globes. C.L. Burns & L.T. Chylack Jr., (1979) Ann. Ophthal. **11:**1358-1368.

Treatment of burns. J.S. Cason, (1981); published by Chapman & Hall.

Practical aspects of wound dressings. A.R. Groves, (1982) Wound healing symposium, pp. 129-136, Ed. J.C. Lawrence; published by the Medicine Publishing Foundation.

Ocular flora in the severely burned patient. C. Pramhus, T.E. Runyan & R.B. Lindberg, (1978) Arch. Ophthal. **96:**1421-1424.

Cicatricial upper lid entropion treated with banked scleral graft. R.R. Tenzel, G.R. Miller & R. Rubenzik, (1975) Arch. Ophthalmol. **93:**999-1000.

Repair and reconstruction in the orbital region. J.C. Mustarde, 2nd edn (1980); published by Churchill Livingstone.

A manual of systematic eyelid surgery. J.R.O. Collin, (1982); published by Churchill Livingstone.

Chapter 5

Ocular damage after blunt trauma to the eye. Its relationship to the nature of the injury. E.M. Eagling, (1974) Brit. J. Ophthal. **58:**126-140.

Traumatic hyphema. W. Rakusin, (1972) Amer. J. Ophthal. **74:**284-292.

Iridectomy in the surgical management of Eight-ball hyphema. R. Parrish & V. Bernardino Jr., (1982) Arch. Ophthalmol. **100:**435-437.

Anterior segment applications of vitrectomy techniques. R.G. Michels, (1978) Trans. Ophthal. Soc. U.K. **98:**458-465.

Gonioscopy in traumatic hyphema. A.M. Tonjum, (1966) Acta Ophthalmol. **44:**650-664.

Anterior chamber angle tears after non-perforating injury. D. Mooney, (1972) Brit. J. Ophthal. **56:**418-424.

Glaucoma after traumatic angle recession. J.H. Kaufman & D.W. Tolpin, (1974) Amer. J. Ophthal. **78:**648-654.

Traumatic haemorrhagic detachment of retinal pigment epithelium. K.A. Gitter, M. Slusher & J. Justice Jr., (1968) Arch. Ophthalmol. **79:**729-732.

Indirect choroidal tears at the posterior pole: a fluorescein angiographic and perimetric study. J.C.D. Hart, V.E. Natsikos, E.R. Raistrick & R.M.L. Doran, (1980) Brit. J. Ophthal. **64:**59-67.

Peripheral fundus changes associated with ocular contusion. D.T. Weidenthal & C.L. Schepens, (1966) Amer. J. Ophthal. **62:**465-477.

Retinal detachment due to ocular contusion. M.S. Cox, C.L. Schepens & H.M. Freeman, (1966) Arch. Ophthal. (Chicago) **76:**678-685.

Complete avulsion of the optic nerve. A clinical, angiographic and electrodiagnostic study. J.S. Hillman, V. Myska & S. Nissim, (1975) Brit. J. Ophthal. **59:**503-509.

Chapter 6

Perforating Eye Injuries (see also references for Chapters 8 and 9)

The treatment of ocular injuries. M.J. Roper-Hall, (1959) Trans. Ophthal. Soc. U.K. **80:**57-69.

A retrospective study of eye injuries. M.J. Roper-Hall, (1969) Ophthalmologica **158:**12-27.

Perforating eye injuries: a five-year survey. S. Johnston, (1971) Trans. Ophthal. Soc. U.K. **91:**895-921.

Vitrectomy in intraocular trauma: its rationale, and its indications and limitations. W.H. Coles & G.M. Haik, (1972) Arch. Ophthalmol. **87:**621-628.

Perforating injuries involving the posterior segment. E.M. Eagling, (1975) Trans. Ophthal. Soc. U.K. **95:**335-339.

Perforating injuries of the eye. E.M. Eagling, (1976) Brit. J. Ophthal. **60:**732-736.

Electrodiagnosis and ultrasonography in the assessment of recent major trauma. S.J. Crews, J.S. Hillman & C.R.S. Thompson, (1975) Brit. J. Ophthal. **95:**315-321.

Primary vitrectomy as a preventive surgical procedure in the treatment of severely injured eyes. J. Faulborn, A. Atkinson & D. Olivier, (1977) Brit. J. Ophthal. **61:**202-208.

Management of trauma of the anterior segment. H. Neubauer, (1978) Trans. Ophthal. Soc. U.K. **98:**30-33.

Closed intraocular microsurgery in ocular trauma. J.J. Kanski, (1978) Trans. Ophthal. Soc. U.K. **98:**51-54.

Retinal Detachment due to Ocular Penetration. M.S. Cox & H.M. Freeman, (1978) Arch. Ophthalmol. **96:**1354-1361.

Perforating injuries of cornea and sclera. J.L. Jay, (1982) Trans. Ophthal. Soc. U.K. **102:**218-220.

Immediate management of iris and lens in perforations of the eye. M.J. Roper-Hall, (1982) Trans. Ophthal. Soc. U.K. **102:**221-222.

Immediate management of posterior perforating trauma. R.J. Cooling, (1982) Trans. Ophthal. Soc. U.K. **102:**223-224.

Control of astigmatism after surgery and trauma. M.J. Roper-Hall, (1982) Brit. J. Ophthal. **66:**556-559.

Changes in endothelial cell density following accidental trauma. M.J. Roper-Hall, R.S. Wilson & S.M. Thompson, (1982) Brit. J. Ophthal., **66:**518-519.

Intraocular Foreign Bodies (see also references for Chapter 9)

A decade of intraocular foreign bodies. S.P.B. Percival, (1972) Brit. J. Ophthal. **56:**454-461.

Intraocular copper foreign bodies. A.R. Rosenthal, B. Appleton & J.L. Hopkins, (1974) Amer. J. Ophthal. **78:**671-678.

Intraocular foreign bodies. H. Neubauer, (1975) Trans. Ophthal. Soc. U.K. **95:**496-501.

Surgical management of nonmagnetic intraocular foreign bodies. R.G. Michels, (1975) Arch. Ophthalmol. **93:**1003-1006.

Intraocular foreign bodies: indications for lensectomy and vitrectomy. E. O'Neill & E.M. Eagling, (1978) Trans. Ophthal. Soc. U.K. **98:**47-48.

The radiography of foreign bodies in the eye as carried out at the Birmingham & Midland Eye Hospital. P. Truelove, (1978) Radiography No. 528 **44:**293-296.

Multisection tomography as an aid in the localisation of intraocular foreign bodies. G.A.S. Lloyd, (1973) Brit. J. Radiology **46:**34-37.

Use of electroacoustic localisation in the management of intraocular foreign bodies. G.A. Sutton, (1979) Brit. J. Ophthal. **63:**787-789.

Ocular metallosis. H. Neubauer, (1979) Trans. Ophthal. Soc. U.K. **99:**502-510.

Sympathetic Ophthalmitis & Intraocular Infections

Sympathetic Ophthalmia: a long-term follow-up. T.A. Makley & A. Azar, (1978) Arch. Ophthal. **96:**257-262.

Immunological investigations in post-traumatic granulomatous and non-granulomatous uveitis. A. Rahi, G. Morgan, I. Levy & W. Dinning, (1978) Brit. J. Ophthal. **62:**722-728.

Aetiology of sympathetic ophthalmitis. N.A. Rao & V.G. Wong, (1981) Trans. Ophthal. Soc. U.K. **101:**357-360.

Treatment of suppurative intraocular infections. J.J. Kanski, (1970) Brit. J. Ophthal. **54:**316-322.

Vitrectomy in Endophthalmitis. A.J. Cottingham Jr. & R.K. Forster, (1976) Arch. Ophthalmol. **94:**2078-2081.

Chapter 7

Ultrasound in pre-vitrectomy assessment. M. Restori & D. McLeod, (1977) Trans. Ophthal. Soc. U.K. **97:**232-234.

Ultrasonic examination of the traumatized eye. M. Restori & D. McLeod, (1978) Trans. Ophthal. Soc. U.K. **98**:38-42.

Electrodiagnosis and ultrasonography in the assessment of recent major trauma. S.J. Crews, J.S. Hillman & C.R.S. Thompson, (1975) Trans. Ophthal. Soc. U.K. **95**:315-321.

Electrophysiological and pathological investigation of concussional injury. J.C. Dean Hart, R. Blight, R. Cooper & D. Papakostopoulos, (1975) Trans. Ophthal. Soc. U.K. **95**:326-334.

The E.R.G. and V.E.P. in patients with severe eye injury. S.J. Crews, C.R.S. Thompson & G.F.A. Harding, (1980) Docum. Ophthal. Proc. Series **15**:203-209.

Magnetic orbital implants. A.D. Atkins & M.J. RoperHall, (1983) Brit. J. Ophth. **67**:315-316.

Perforating injuries involving the posterior segment. E.M. Eagling, (1975) Trans. Ophthal. Soc. U.K. **95**:335-339.

Trampolines and triangles: The surgical pathology of the vitreous. D. McLeod & P.K. Leaver, (1977) Trans. Ophthal. Soc. U.K. **97**:225-231.

Vitrectomy in the management of the injured eye. A.J. Atkinson, (1977) Trans. Ophthal. Soc. U.K. **97**:254-255.

Experimental posterior penetrating eye injury in the rabbit. I. Method of production and natural history. II. Histology of wound, vitreous and retina. P.E. Cleary & S.J. Ryan, (1979) Brit. J. Ophth. **63**:306-311; **63**:312-321.

Experimental posterior penetrating eye injury in the rhesus monkey: vitreous-lens admixture. P.E. Cleary, G. Jarus & S.J. Ryan, (1980) Brit. J. Ophth. **64**:801-808.

Penetrating eye injuries: a histopathological review. S.R. Winthrop, P.E. Cleary, D.S. Minckler & S.J. Ryan, (1980) Brit. J. Ophth. **64**:809-817.

Combined posterior contusion and penetrating injury in the pig eye. I. A natural history study. II. Histological features. Z. Gregor & J. Ryan, (1982) Brit. J. Ophth. **66**:793-798; **66**:799-804.

Treatment of major trauma of the anterior segment. H. Neubauer, (1975) Trans. Ophthal. Soc. U.K. **95**:322-325.

The management of anterior segment trauma with multiple small incisions. R.H. Keates & S.B. Lichtenstein, (1980) Ophthalmology Philadelphia **87**:887-891.

Vitreous surgery techniques in penetrating ocular trauma. R.G. Michels & B.P. Conway, (1978) Trans. Ophthal. Soc. U.K. **98**:472-480.

Sympathetic uveitis and phakoanaphylaxis. J.C. Allen, (1967) Am. J. Ophthalmol. **63**:280-283.

Sympathetic ophthalmitis treated with azathioprine. C.E. Moore, (1968) Brit. J. Ophth. **52**:688-690.

Clinically unsuspected phakoanaphylaxis after ocular trauma. E.M. Perlman & D.M. Albert, (1977) Arch. Ophthal. **95**:244-246.

Vogt-Koyanagi-Harada syndrome. S. Ohno, D.H. Char, S.J. Kimura & G.R. O'Connor, (1977) Am. J. Ophthalmol. **83**:735-740.

Sympathetic Ophthalmia: a long-term follow-up. T.A. Makley Jr. & A. Azar, (1978) Arch. Ophthal. **96**:257-262.

Immunological investigations in post-traumatic granulomatous and non-granulomatous uveitis. A. Rahi, G. Morgan, I. Levy & W. Dinning, (1978) Brit. J. Ophthal. **62**:722-728.

Pigmentation-associated histopathological variations in sympathetic ophthalmia. G.E. Marak & H. Ikui, (1980) Brit. J. Ophth. **64**:220-222.

Aetiology of sympathetic ophthalmitis. N.A. Rao & V.G. Wong, (1981) Trans. Ophthal. Soc. U.K. **101**:357-360.

The treatment of suppurative intraocular infections. J.J. Kanski, (1970) Brit. J. Ophthal. **54**:316-322.

Endophthalmitis: diagnostic cultures and results. R.K. Forster, (1974) Arch. Ophthalmol. **92**:387-392.

Clinical use of intravitreal antibiotics to treat bacterial endophthalmitis. G.A. Peyman, D.W. Vastine, E.R. Crouch & R.W. Herbst Jr., (1974) Trans. Am. Acad. Ophthalmol. Otolaryngol. **78**:862-875.

Vitrectomy in endophthalmitis. A.J. Cottingham Jr. & R.K. Forster, (1976) Arch. Ophthalmol. **94**:2078-2081.

Chapter 8

Microsurgical control of corneal astigmatism in cataract and keratoplasty. R.C. Troutman, (1973) Trans. Amer. Acad. Ophthalmol. Otolaryngol. **77**:563-572.

Perforating injuries of the eye. E.M. Eagling, (1976) Brit. J. Ophthal. **60**:732-736.

Repair of corneal wounds and the elimination of astigmatism. R.C. Troutman, (1978) Trans. Ophthal. Soc. U.K. **98**:49-50.

Surgical correction of high postkeratoplasty astigmatism. J.H. Krachmer & R.E. Fenzl, (1980) Arch. Ophthalmol. **98**:1400-1402.

Control of astigmatism after surgery and trauma. M.J. Roper-Hall, (1982) Brit. J. Ophthal. **66**:556-559.

Control of astigmatism after surgery and trauma: a new technique. M.J. Roper-Hall & D. Atkins, (1985) Brit. J. Ophthal. **69**:352-359.

Reduction in endothelial cell density following cataract extraction and intraocular lens implantation. M.J. Roper-Hall & R.S. Wilson, (1982) Brit. J. Ophthal. **66**:516-517.

Changes in endothelial cell density following accidental trauma. M.J. Roper-Hall, R.S. Wilson & S.M. Thompson, (1982) Brit. J. Ophthal. **66**:518-519.

Visco-elastic materials in the surgery of ocular trauma. M.J. Roper-Hall, (1983) Trans. Ophthal. Soc. U.K. **103**:274-276.

Corneal transplantation for severe alkali burns. S.I. Brown, M.P. Tragakis & D.B. Pearce, (1972) Trans. Amer. Acad. Ophthalmol. Otolaryngol. **76**:1266-1274.

Anterior segment surgery early after corneal wound repair. E. Maul & R. Muga, (1977) Brit. J. Ophthal. **61**:782-784.

Management of trauma of the anterior segment. H. Neubauer, (1978) Trans. Ophthal. Soc. U.K. **98**:30-33.

The management of anterior segment trauma with multiple small incisions. R.H. Keates & S.B. Lichtenstein, (1980) Ophthalmology Philadelphia **87**:887-891.

Traumatic cataract. M.J. Roper-Hall, (1977) Trans. Ophthal. Soc. U.K. **97**:58-59.

Secondary reconstruction. M.J. Roper-Hall, (1975) Trans. Ophthal. Soc. U.K. **95**:346-348.

Keratoprosthesis: a long-term review. J.J. Barnham & M.J. Roper-Hall, (1983) Brit. J. Ophthal. **67**:468-474.

One hundred consecutive pars plana vitrectomies using the vitreophage. G.A. Peyman, F.V. Huamonte & M.F. Goldberg, (1976) Finer J. Ophthal. **81**:263-271.

Chapter 9

Perforating injuries involving the posterior segment. E.M. Eagling, (1975) Trans. Ophthal. Soc. U.K. **95:**335-339.

Intraocular foreign bodies: indications for lensectomy and vitrectomy. E. O'Neill & E.M. Eagling, (1978) Trans. Ophthal. Soc. U.K. **98:**47-48.

Guidelines in the management of penetrating ocular trauma with the emphasis on the role and timing of pars plana vitrectomy. S.J. Ryan, (1979) Int. Ophthal. **1:**105-108.

Closed microsurgery in the management of intraocular foreign bodies. R.J. Cooling, D. McLeod, R.K. Blach & P.K. Leaver, (1981) Trans. Ophthalmol. Soc. U.K. **101:**181-183.

Surgical management of non-magnetic intraocular foreign bodies. R.G. Michels, (1975) Arch. Ophthalmol. **93:**1003-1006.

Ocular metallosis. H. Neubauer, (1979) Trans. Ophthal. Soc. U.K. **99:**502-510.

Giant tear of the retina. J.D. Scott, (1975) Trans. Ophthal. Soc. U.K. **95:**142-144.

Vitrectomy and fluid/silicone-oil exchange for giant retinal tears: results at six months. P.K. Leaver, R.J. Cooling, E.B. Feretis, J.S. Lean & D. McLeod, (1984) Brit. J. Ophthal. **68:**432-438.

The use of Lincoff balloons in the management of retinal detachment. T. Fetherston & E.M. Eagling, (1982) Trans. Ophthal. Soc. U.K. **102:**230-232.

Chapter 10

Repair and reconstruction in the orbital region. J.C. Mustarde, (1980) Churchill Livingstone, 2nd edn.

A manual of systematic eyelid surgery. J.R.O. Collin, (1983) Churchill Livingstone.

Long-term review of injuries to the lacrimal apparatus. Y.M. Canavan & D.B. Archer, (1979) Trans. Ophthal. Soc. U.K. **99:**201-204.

Naso-orbital fractures, complications and treatment. C.K. Beyer, R.L. Fabian & B. Smith, (1982) Ophthalmology **89:**456-463.

Maxillofacial Injuries. Ed. N.L. Rowe & J.L. Williams, (1985) Churchill Livingstone.

The natural and unnatural history of a blow-out fracture. E. Waddell, P. Fells & L. Koornneeff, (1982) Brit. Orthopt. J. **39:**29-32.

Paresis and restriction of the inferior rectus muscle after orbital floor fracture. B.J. Kushner, (1982) Amer. J. Ophthalmol. **94:**81-86.

Adjustable strabismus surgical procedures. A. Jampolsky, (1978) p. 321 Trans. of the New Orleans Acad. Ophthalmology.

The use of adjustable sutures. P. Fells, (1981) Trans. Ophthal. Soc. U.K. **101:**279-283.

Traumatic third nerve palsy. J.S. Elston, (1984) Brit. J. Ophthal. **68:**538-543.

Surgical treatment of ptosis in acquired third nerve paralysis. C.K. Beyer & R.W. McCarthy, (1981) Ann. Ophthal. (Chic.) **13:**373-376.

Management of large angle exotropia. J.H. Goldstein & J. Freeman, (1978) Ann. Ophthal. (Chic.) **10:**1739-1744.

Rectus muscle union in sixth nerve paralysis. B.R. Frueh & J.W. Henderson, (1971) Arch. Ophthalmol. **85:**191-196.

The Faden operation: when and how to do it. W. de Decker, (1981) Trans. Ophthal. Soc. U.K. **101:**264-270.

The Adjustable Harada-Ito Procedure. H.S. Metz & H. Lerner, (1981) Arch. Ophthalmol. **99:**624-626.

Treatment of unilateral fourth nerve paralysis. P. Knapp, (1981) Trans. Ophthal. Soc. U.K. **101:**273-275.

Blindness from accident. Ed. J.F. Cullen (1976) for the W.H. Ross Foundation.

Index